Practical Approaches to Infection Control in Residential Aged Care

Second Edition

THIS BOOK HAS BEEN ENDORSED BY
ROYAL COLLEGE OF NURSING, AUSTRALIA
ACCORDING TO APPROVED CRITERIA

Ausmed Publications
Selected Titles

Practical Approaches to Infection Control in Residential Aged Care

Second Edition

By Kevin J. Kendall

Foreword by Sue Cornish

AUSMED PUBLICATIONS PTY LTD
MELBOURNE, AUSTRALIA

Ausmed Publications Pty Ltd
277 Mt Alexander Road, Ascot Vale,
Melbourne, Victoria 3032, Australia
ABN 49 824 739 129
Telephone: + 61 3 9375 7311
Fax: + 61 3 9375 7299
E-mail: ausmed@ausmed.com.au
<www.ausmed.com.au>

Although the Publisher has taken every care to ensure the accuracy of the professional, clinical and technical components of this publication, it accepts no responsibility for any loss or damage suffered by any person as a result of following the procedures described or acting on information set out in this publication. The Publisher reminds readers that the information in this publication is no substitute for individual medical and/or nursing assessment and treatment by professional staff.

First published by Ausmed Publications Pty Ltd. in 1998, second edition 2003.
All rights reserved.

National Library of Australia Cataloguing-in-Publication data:
Kendall, Kevin. J (Kevin James), 1951—.
Practical approaches to infection control in residential aged care.
2nd edition
Bibliography.
Includes index.
ISBN: 0 9579876 0 9

1. Communicable diseases in old age—Prevention. 2. Aged—Institutional care.
3. Aged—health and hygiene. 4. Old age homes—Health aspects. I. Title.
618.9769

Edited by Trisha Dunning
Printed in Australia

Acknowledgments

For helpful comments on an earlier version of this material:

Dr Peter Arndt, Miss Lorna Chapman, Ms Jill Clutterbuck, Ms Catherine Evans, Mr Brian Fitzpatrick, Ms Annette Hicks, Ms Helen Goble, Mr Simon Lam, Ms Jillian Macloy, Ms Bronwen Mander, Ms Prue Mellor, Mr Rodney Moran, Ms Catherine Peerman, Ms Julie Reed, Mr Tony Stacey, Ms Lyn Wight, Mr Rory Wilby, Dr Maria Yates.

For advice:

Media Unit of the Victorian Department of Human Services

Contents

List of figures and tables

Foreword

Aged care is an ever-growing field with an increasing number of people over 65 years of age. Many aged people need supported care within hostels or nursing homes both now and in the immediate future. With the reduction of stay in the acute-care sector, many aged residents return to residential accommodation requiring a substantial amount of support and care. They also have the possibility of returning to the accommodation carrying antibiotic-resistant organisms. Because of reduced immunity, aged people are very vulnerable to infections. Residence within an aged-care facility now carries the same risks for the acquisition of nosocomial infections as in the acute-care sector. Therefore, greater effort is required to avoid unnecessary infections in residents of aged-care facilities.

The need to understand infection-control requirements within the residential aged-care sector is of the utmost importance for the residents and staff of such facilities. The stringent application of infection-control principles and practice is imperative in reducing the number of nosocomial infections in residents in long-term care. The Accreditation Standards recognise this in their requirements for aged-care facilities. However, there is a dearth of information in this area. This volume addresses the need for information on infection control within the aged health-care sector. The demand for such information is reflected in this, the second edition of Kevin Kendall's book.

Kevin Kendall has extensive experience in infection control, culminating in the position of clinical nurse consultant at Fairfield Infectious Diseases Hospital before its redistribution and closure. Over his career he has also worked for many years within the aged-care sector. His extensive experience in infection control and aged care has given him a unique opportunity to marry these two areas of expertise. This volume is testament to that knowledge and expertise. Kevin's approach is straightforward and practical, and therefore has appeal and application to a broad audience. This has great value within the aged-care sector as it involves people from disparate backgrounds and knowledge bases. Therefore, this volume is a great resource for all those who are employed in the care of residents within the aged-care sector.

Kevin continues to advance his knowledge and experience in infection control and aged care, and is a valued lecturer and resource in this area. The need for information in infection control in residential aged care will only increase, and this volume is valued for its timeliness and practicality in a rapidly growing area of health care.

Susan Cornish

Course Coordinator/Lecturer

Infection Control and Sterilisation

Mayfield Education Centre

Introduction

Introduction

We are all at risk of acquiring infections. Every hour of every day we come into contact with potentially harmful micro-organisms—on the hands we shake in friendship, from the coffee cups at work, or even in the potting mixes we use in the garden. Serious illness is usually avoided because our defence mechanisms work efficiently. Our skin is strong and intact, our circulation is efficient, and we produce mature white blood cells in adequate numbers. However, the residents in our care at work might not be so well protected.

This book is written to assist nurses and other care providers to reduce the risk of transmitting infection from:

- staff to residents or visitors;
- resident to resident;
- resident to staff members or visitors; and
- staff member to staff member.

People of all ages admitted to hospitals and residential-care facilities are more likely to succumb to the harmful effects of micro-organisms in the immediate environment.[1,2] Older people are at great risk of infection due to the resistance-lowering effects of ageing caused by:

- fragile skin and mucous membranes;
- a less-efficient circulatory system;
- reduced mobility;
- loss of self-caring ability;
- onset of chronic disease (such as type 2 diabetes mellitus); and
- malignancies and their treatment.

Experience has shown that the residents most vulnerable to infection are those who require the greatest amount of care from staff. As well as elderly residents, this includes the growing group of younger, disabled residents living in aged-care facilities. Unfortunately, apart from anecdotal evidence, there are little data available to identify actual infection statistics in residential facilities.

4
Infection Control

Infections acquired in the course of care (nosocomial infections) will, at the least, cause discomfort and increase costs. However, they can also markedly reduce an individual's quality of life, and can even lead to death. Nosocomial infections among staff members increase compensable work-related illness and sick leave, and resident infections can significantly increase the cost of care. At a time when health-care costs are under constant review, these factors have implications for all who work in residential facilities.

Residential care staff must be educated and ready to manage the infection-control risks of a higher level of care for frailer, sicker residents.

The trend in aged care is for elderly people to be maintained in the community until they are very dependent. Residential care staff must now be competent to protect an increasingly frail group of residents against acquired and preventable infections, while maintaining the individual resident's privacy and dignity.[3] In the future, if such frail residents need acute treatment for severe infection, they might be treated in the residential facility rather than being transferred to an acute facility. In the context of economically driven changes to the health-care system and the needs of the individual resident, there is much that staff and management can do to ensure effective infection control. In practical terms, the following strategies might form basic components of an overall infection control approach:

- careful admission history-taking that includes enquiring about the new resident's infectious diseases history; if the resident is confused, relatives and friends might also be a source of information;
- planned strategies to prevent the transmission of infection—including offering residents and staff an annual influenza vaccination and residents a pneumococcal vaccination every ten years;
- a person with an interest and, preferably, formal education in infection-control procedures maintaining the facility's infection control program;
- an active infection-control committee meeting regularly to: (i) review statistical information, results of audits and quality activities; and (ii) consider matters of concern; alternatively, infection control could be a subcommittee or a permanent agenda item of another committee (for example, an occupational health-and-safety committee).

Infection control education includes:

- orientating all staff to the infection-control implications of their various roles;
- acquainting new staff with the facility's infection-control policies and practices;
- providing ongoing infection-control education for all staff, at all levels, at least annually;
- regularly bathing and worming pets that live at or visit the facility and keeping them free of fleas; and
- external service providers (such as caterers, butchers, laundry services, podiatrists, hairdressers, gardeners and waste-collectors) being contracted on the basis of their satisfactory compliance with recommended infection-control standards and practices, specific to their area of operation.

Infection control is only as strong as each part of the facility's strategy. It is therefore vital that each staff member takes responsibility for his or her own actions in the workplace. To maintain good infection-control practices, staff must assess the possibility of exposure to body fluids and other infection risks. This should occur during each interaction with residents, and staff members should be taking any protective precautions that are necessary. The level of infection in any facility is an important measure of quality of care. It is, therefore, imperative that effective infection-control strategies and monitoring programs be established and supported by both management and staff.

After more than a decade, the Commonwealth Outcome Standards for residential care have been reviewed. Although infection control is a component of all four revised standards and their expected outcomes, it is specifically addressed in Standard 4, *Physical Environment and Safe Systems*, which is divided into:

- Infection Control (Standard 4.7)
- Catering, Cleaning and Laundry Service (Standard 4.8).[4]

The expected outcomes of these standards (required for accreditation purposes) demand that facility management can demonstrate:

- continuous improvement of care;
- regulatory compliance;
- education and staff development programs and strategies.[5]

The standards are deliberately general so they can be applied to the wide variety of situations found among individual residents and facilities. This book will assist both direct carers and management to establish, implement, and maintain practices that comply with the standards. The book will also be a useful reference for those who monitor and audit compliance with government standards.

6
Infection Control

The book will not provide a foolproof formula for meeting the standards and regulations concerned with infection control. However, it will provide: (i) *residential care staff* with a sound basis for decision-making about how to best care for residents and themselves; (ii) *management* with the background information necessary to safeguard staff and residents and (iii) *ancillary staff* with solid guidelines about how to do their jobs safely.

The interaction among residents, visitors, and staff is at the heart of care. The context of care is the inanimate environment—not only the building, plant, and equipment, but also the management policies and practices. Standards and regulations are met by considering all these aspects, not by following a recipe. Whether a facility is comprised of 30 beds or 200 beds, whether the building is old or new, and whether it is stand-alone or attached to a large health service, the care of residents should be the same. It should not be compromised, and it should be acceptable to what carers would wish for their own relatives and for themselves if ever they were admitted.

Judging by the response to the first edition of this popular textbook, the second edition (with updated information) will be welcomed by nurses and other care workers in residential aged-care settings. The duty of care owed to elderly, frail residents by carers includes the prevention, source identification, and management of infections. Contemporary professional standards set the framework for these activities.

The aim of the second edition of this book is to convey current information to ensure a match between practice standards and the everyday reality of trying to protect residents and staff from infection. As well, there is new information for the reader—such as additional tables and figures.

The book has seven distinct, but overlapping, chapters. Before beginning the chapters, readers can test themselves with the 'Frequently Asked Questions' (p. 7)—and can check the answers at the end of the book. There is also a comprehensive glossary at the end of the book.

Since this book was written, severe acute respiratory syndrome (SARS) has been identified and classified as a notifiable disease in Australia.

Frequently Asked Questions

Frequently asked questions

Confusion abounds about the source, transmission, and treatment of infection. People fear that they might contract an infection in the workplace or at home. Often such unnecessary fears can be dispelled by information or advice from a qualified person, such as a health worker.

Health-care workers have a duty to keep their knowledge up to date. They are then in a good position to care for their residents, and to inform others about infection control. Sadly, there is still a great deal of ignorance about infection control, even among health carers. When others express ignorance-based fears about infection, take the opportunity to pass on a little of the knowledge you will gain from this book—an informed community is a safer community.

Test yourself with these questions. You might be surprised at how little, or how much, you know. The answers can be found on pages 161–7.

1. *My husband is going to have major surgery in a big public hospital. Is he likely to get 'golden staph' while he is there?*

2. *I've heard there are bugs in hospitals now that eat your flesh. How long until they get into aged care?*

3. *Can HIV be transmitted by mosquitoes?*

4. *Can I catch HIV from a door handle touched by a homosexual?*

5. *Is chickenpox a sexually transmitted disease?*

6. *Is it true that shingles causes chickenpox?*

7. *The lady in the next unit has chickenpox. To be safe, how many times do I have to wash my clothes after she has used our washing machine?*

8. *My son lives in the city and has been diagnosed with scabies. He is coming home and has not been treated. Are we at risk in the country?*

9. *One of the laundry staff caught scabies from a resident. Does that mean she wasn't washing her hands properly?*

10. *A resident transported in the centre's car has been diagnosed with head lice, what do we do with the car?*

11. *Can I catch meningitis from a friend at home and then take it to work?*

12. *My doctor has just told me on the telephone that I am a hepatitis B carrier and to see him in three months. What do I do in the meantime, especially about my husband and children?*

13. *My doctor told me I was a hepatitis B carrier and that I should not even shake hands with anybody. Is this correct?*

14. *A person with hepatitis C has slashed himself. What do I do with the knife?*

15. *A person in the hostel room next to me has hepatitis C. How can I get him out of the hostel?*

16. *A friend who I think has HIV washes his Band-Aids prior to disposal. Is that right?*

17. *I needed a fix yesterday and the only syringe and needle available were from an HIV positive person. Do you think I will get it?*

18. *I want a tattoo. Can I catch HIV this way?*

19. *I have bought a second-hand thermos and my husband is afraid of catching AIDS from it. Is this possible?*

20. *I'm HIV positive, do I have to tell my employer?*

21. *We want to screen all our new residents for hepatitis B, hepatitis C, and HIV—just so we know if any of them are infectious. What do you think?*

22. *The charge nurse says we have to use 'university precautions' when we empty pans. I left school before VCE so does it apply to me?*

23. *At our establishment we practice standard precautions, but what do we do with the linen now we have a hepatitis B carrier as a resident?*

24. *We have admitted our first HIV resident. Is it appropriate to use disposable cutlery and crockery?*

25. *One of our residents is 79 and used to be gay. Should we test him for HIV?*

26. *Our establishment has been asked to admit an elderly woman who is HIV positive. I am not worried about the HIV but have grave concerns about the AIDS.*

27. *Our occupational health and safety policy states that AIDS can be transmitted through unbroken skin and is very virulent this way. Is this correct?*

28. *Is it true that all linen skips should be covered with drawsheets to keep the bugs in?*

29. *In our nursing home, the staff wear long-sleeved gowns and gloves all day, to ensure that no staff members are placed at risk of acquiring any infection. Is this appropriate?*

30. *We are a nursing home and all our patients are clean. Do we really need infection-control practices in place?*

31. *Is it true that vinegar and methylated spirits are alternatives to disinfectants?*

32. *Is it appropriate to clean bench tops by spraying and wiping with gluteraldehyde?*

33. One of our residents has 'golden staph' in a foot ulcer so we are reverse barrier nursing him in a two-bed room. The staff wear gown, gloves and mask. Is this appropriate?

34. In our establishment we soak all pans in Detsol or Safsol before the sanitiser cycle, just to make sure they are clean. Is this appropriate?

35. Is it satisfactory to put instruments through a hot water disinfector then leave them soaking in sodium hypochlorite until they are required for use?

36. Why is it that recapping of used needles is not recommended?

37. Can we use a microwave oven as a steriliser?

38. I don't know how long to leave the autoclave on for. Can you advise?

39. Is it acceptable to seal steriliser bags with autoclave tape?

40. I get dermatitis from soap. Is it all right if I don't wash my hands before doing a dressing?

41. A patient in the next building had TB. Should I have a chest X-ray?

42. To save on catheter bags the night staff leave catheters draining into urinals. Is that OK?

43. The manager says we have to re-use single-use insulin syringes. We wash them in hot soapy water but I still don't feel right about it. What do you think?

44. We're supposed to wear goggles when sluicing linen, but I don't because some of the staff are gay and I'm worried about catching something. What do you suggest?

45. We soak all the enteral feeding giving sets together in sodium hypochlorite. Is that enough to kill the germs?

46. The labels have come off all the drums in the cleaners' room and I washed the floor with shampoo by mistake. Will it kill the germs anyway?

47. The unit manager says we have to wipe everything with bleach, but it's taking the colour out of the furnishings. Is there an alternative?

48. I'm too short to reach the high shelves with my duster. Is it that important?

49. When the linen is delivered it's still damp. The laundry contractor dumps it on the ground outside the kitchen. Should we make him bring it into the foyer?

50. Why can't we use Betadine packs on wound cavities any more? They used to work well.

12
Infection Control

51. *The union says it's not my job to bring the milk inside when it's delivered to our nursing home. The residents like it warm anyway. Is that a problem?*

52. *We throw all the rubbish in to the skip. The residents in the room beside it complain about the smell, but will they catch anything from it?*

53. *On week nights I have to clean the pan room before I give out the suppers. Is this acceptable?*

54. *We got a new air conditioning system last summer and now every one is getting colds. Could it be Legionnaire's disease?*

55. *There are lots of stray cats behind the hostel, and the kitchen staff leave milk out for them. Will any germs get into the food?*

56. *We had an outbreak of gastroenteritis at work last winter, and even the staff became sick. The DON said it couldn't be the food because the kitchen staff are very clean. Would this be right?*

Once you have read this book you should be able to answer these questions. The answers are on pages 161–7.

Chapter 1

Infection Control Overview

Infection control aims and objectives

Effective infection control is a basic and essential component of the safe environment of care. Every residential facility has a duty of care, or formal obligation, to provide a safe environment for:

- staff;
- residents; and
- visitors.

Although infection control is always the shared concern of management and staff, responsibility for effective infection control starts with management. The facility mission statement should reflect infection control through health promotion, education, and prevention. In order to meet this obligation, management must consult with staff to formulate the infection-control aims and objectives that form the foundation of the facility's infection-control program.

Infection control aims

In order to maintain effective infection control, facility management should:

- institute appropriate measures to prevent transmission of infection between residents, staff, and visitors;
- maintain adequate physical facilities and equipment to control the spread of harmful organisms;
- maintain surveillance systems to detect infections spreading among residents and/or staff;
- implement a course of management and intervention (if a cluster of infections is identified);
- inform staff of any infectious hazards they could face in the course of their employment;
- provide staff with adequate education, resources, and information about hygiene and infection-control practices; and
- use the facility newsletter as a medium for imparting information about infection-control issues to residents, relatives, visitors, and staff.

Infection control objectives

In order to meet the infection-control aims, facility management will:

- identify and address areas 'at risk' in relation to infections;
- formulate, implement, and regularly review infection-control policies and procedures;

- ensure that staff members are consulted and are able to participate in identifying hazards, assessing risks, and developing policies and procedures within the facility;
- ensure, by educational programs, that all levels and classifications of staff are acquainted with, and understand the basis for, the facility's infection-control policies and procedures;
- ensure that all food services staff members carry out appropriate hygiene practices;
- oversee a high standard of cleaning and laundering practices, regularly reviewed to ensure the methods used are up-to-date and efficient;
- provide a hygienic working environment for residents and staff, through sanitation programs and practices;
- adopt a 'standard precautions policy' that establishes that all people in the facility (resident, staff or visitor) might be a potential source of infection;
- ensure that infection control, risk assessment, and quality control are specifically identified in staff position descriptions; and
- institute an 'infection-control surveillance program' that monitors and documents appropriate outcome measures, staff practices, and the incidence of infections among staff and residents.

Much of the content of these aims and objectives will be examined in greater detail in the following pages.

Principles of infection control

The principles of infection control are:

- implementation of various precautionary measures aimed at preventing the occurrence or transmission of infection;
- appreciation of basic microbiology and modes of disease transmission;
- implementation of work practices that prevent transmission of infection;
- conscientious staff hygiene and regular cleaning of work areas, equipment and disinfection;
- adoption of nationally recognised procedures for sterilisation and disinfection;
- modification of clinical procedures that might be affected by or affect an underlying disease, and consideration of alternative, non-invasive procedures;
- routine utilisation of single-use equipment (where practical) and appropriate selection of equipment and supplies.

- appropriate use of antibiotics;
- support for occupational health and safety policy and practices;
- vaccination against infections that are a potential risk in the health-care setting;
- surveillance of nosocomial/iatrogenic and occupationally acquired infections;
- ongoing quality-management and quality-improvement activities;
- legal and ethical considerations;
- ongoing education and training to the appropriate level;
- facility-wide application;
- integration into comprehensive quality-management programs;
- total organisational commitment; and
- regular evaluation of effectiveness (*Infection Control in the Health Care Setting*, April 1996, p. 12).

Source, transmission, and spread of infection

Infection remains a common cause of human disease. It is generally acknowledged worldwide that people admitted to hospital are at risk of acquiring a potentially serious infection. In Australia, it is estimated that 5–10 per cent of patients will acquire a nosocomial infection.[1] Although the types of infections acquired in residential facilities are often less severe than those acquired in major hospitals, they can still have a devastating effect on residents' health and quality of life.

A comprehensive infection-control program will reduce resident-acquired and staff-acquired infections within the facility.[2] Many aged-care facilities are in the process of developing systems to collect statistical information on infections. It is therefore difficult to assess infection rates in aged care at present.

Due to the adaptability of micro-organisms, and their relationship with human hosts, low (but persistent) levels of infectious agents will always be present in human communities. A considerable proportion of residents admitted to a facility will acquire some kind of clinical infection during their stay. The cause, frequency, and severity of infections will vary, and sometimes they are due to definable causes (such as the medical condition of the resident). However, sometimes, for unknown reasons:

- there is an increase in the commonly occurring types of infections/infestations (e.g., influenza and scabies); and
- types of infection appear that are not normally present in the facility (e.g., *Salmonella* infection).

If infection-control practices break down in a facility, the rate of infection and variety of bacteria present will increase, as will the infection risk for staff, residents, and visitors.

Elements in the transmission of infection

For infection to spread in residential care facilities, or any human community, four elements are necessary. These form the 'chain of infection' (see Figure 1.1): They are:

- the presence of pathogenic or disease-producing micro-organisms, surviving in a reservoir;
- exit of the disease-producing micro-organisms from the reservoir;
- the means of transmission of the disease-producing micro-organisms; and
- entry of micro-organisms into susceptible people, or hosts, who then develop an infection and/or an infectious disease and can themselves become a reservoir or source of infection.

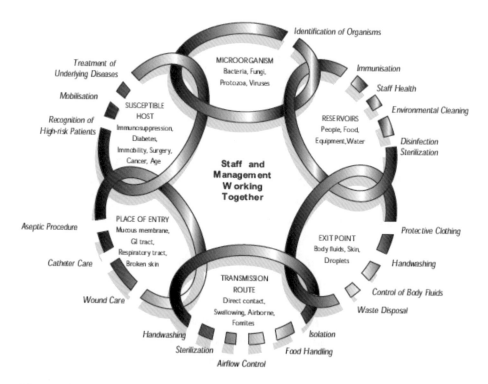

Figure 1.
The chain of infection CAN be broken.

When staff understand the factors that contribute to the cyclical process of the chain of infection, intervention is possible, and the chain can be broken by good infection-control work practices.

1. Pathogens in a reservoir

The pathogens (disease-causing micro-organisms) in a reservoir range from large, complex protozoa to ultramicroscopic viruses. Larger parasites (such as worms, mites, and lice) can also cause disease. Some agents that infect humans are yet to be identified.

Infections acquired in the community are more commonly caused by bacteria, such as *Staphylococcus aureus*, *Streptococcus pyogenes*, and *Salmonella* species. Types of pathogenic viruses include the well-known measles, mumps, varicella (chicken pox) and herpes viruses.

Any organism acquired by residents, staff, or visitors can cause infections in residential facilities. However, the ability of the micro-organism to cause infection depends on:

- the resident's own defence mechanisms;
- the ability of the micro-organism to cause disease (pathogenicity); and
- the number of that type of micro-organisms present (the degree of contamination).

Some particular pathogenic organisms are closely associated with institutional infections—for example, *Escherichia coli* (*E. coli*). Relatively harmless micro-organisms can become pathogenic in residential facilities because residents' defences are often reduced. Such opportunistic organisms normally colonise residents' own bodies (normal flora) without causing illness, but become pathogenic when residents are susceptible.

Opportunistic organisms (e.g., *Pseudomonas* or *Staphylococcus*) can become resistant to many antibiotics and are able to flourish in conditions under which most disease-producing organisms cannot multiply. Well-known examples include the so-called 'super bugs'—for example, methicillin-resistant *Staphylococcus aureus* (MRSA) and vancomycin-resistant *Enterococcus* (VRE). As reported in the press from time-to-time, hospital patients are increasingly exposed to these 'super bugs' that can pose a great risk to health and life in susceptible individuals.

Antibiotic-resistant organisms develop as the result of:

- inappropriate use, or over-prescribing, of antibiotics;
- failure to complete a prescribed course of antibiotics; and
- inappropriate use of disinfectants for cleaning.

Reservoirs include humans, animals, or the inanimate environment.[3] Human reservoirs of infection include people who are temporarily ill with an infectious disease, or people who are long-term carriers of organisms. Similarly, animals can act as reservoirs for pathogens that are transmissible to humans or other animals. Under favourable conditions, reservoirs of pathogens can develop within a building or in a garden.

Specific examples of reservoirs of infection in a facility include:

- residents or staff who have an infectious disease (such as influenza);
- residents or staff who are carriers of hepatitis B;
- residents returning from hospital colonised by pathogens;
- visitors to the facility who have an infection;
- pets infested with parasites; and
- contaminated water in cooling towers or shower heads.

In general, high-risk reservoirs of infection are those in which bacteria can readily multiply. Because organisms cannot multiply on dry objects or surfaces such as workbenches (although they can survive there), septic wounds are more likely to be a higher-risk source of infection.

2. Exit of the disease-producing micro-organisms from the reservoir

When disease-producing micro-organisms leave the reservoir, spread of infection is likely to occur. Organisms leave a human reservoir via infected body fluids—such as droplets of saliva or sputum (when the infected person coughs). Staff members have an opportunity to break the chain at the point where bacteria leave the reservoir, simply by maintaining good infection-control practices, such as:

- correct hand-washing;
- wearing protective apparel; and
- safe disposal of infected body fluids.

3. The means of transmitting disease-producing micro-organisms

The many ways that micro-organisms can be transmitted will be discussed in greater detail later in this chapter. In terms of the chain of infection, it is sufficient to understand that every form of direct and indirect human contact provides an opportunity for disease-producing micro-organisms to be transmitted. However, hands contaminated with micro-organisms are the most common means of spreading infection.

The next greatest risk of infection transmission is by contact with contaminated equipment used for invasive procedures—for example catheter tips or suturing material. Other means of spread include:

- contaminated food, resulting in outbreaks of gastroenteritis;
- the flow of air currents within the facility spreading a viral infection; and, less frequently
- staff clothing contaminated with organism-containing body fluids.

4. The micro-organism's entry into susceptible people

Humans can become hosts to micro-organisms when normal body defences are compromised. For residents, this can be due to such factors as:

- broken skin or mucous membranes (such as wounds or bed sores) coming into contact with contaminated material;
- inhaling airborne organisms when the cough reflex is absent or diminished (for example, as a result of brain injury);
- undergoing multiple invasive procedures (including urinary catheterisation);
- taking immunosuppressant medications (such as prednisolone); and
- having a concurrent infection.[4]

Route of transmission[5]

Intervention at the point of transmission is an effective way to break the chain of infection. When the route of infection is identified, specific steps can be taken to disrupt transmission. Routes of transmission can be classified as:

1. *Exogenous or external infections*—which have a source outside the body (e.g., another person or the environment), and are spread by: (i) airborne transfer, (ii) direct contact, (iii) common vehicle transmission, or (iv) vectorborne transmission. Exogenous infections are spread by cross infection.
2. *Endogenous or self-infections* develop from the body's normal flora.

1. Exogenous infection

Regardless of the causative organism, cross infection from a resident or member of staff to others can occur by the following routes:

- staff or visitors' hands or clothing;
- ambulant residents touching other people or objects; and
- people using contaminated objects, fluids or food.

Contact transmission is by directly or indirectly touching another person or object. When busy staff members are caring for too many residents, staff can inadvertently contribute to cross-infection by transferring infective organisms from one resident to another, unless strict hygiene is practised.

Airborne transmission can occur when bacteria and viruses are spread by coughing and sneezing. Minute droplets dispersed from the mouth and nose are a potential source of airborne infection, especially at times when respiratory infections are at a peak in the general community. In order to stop infection being transferred by the airborne route:

- infected visitors can be discouraged from visiting;
- residents and staff should be vaccinated against influenza; and
- sick staff should not attend to residents.

Common vehicle transmission occurs when a person becomes infected after contact with a contaminated product, such as contaminated blood, medication, food or water.

Animals or insects spread *vectorborne pathogens*—for example when flies spread micro-organisms.

2. Endogenous infection

Self-infection is a hazard for residents whose immune systems are compromised. As already discussed, such residents are at risk of their body flora acting pathogenically at a body site not normally colonised by the organism. Common organisms of self-infection, and their usual body sites, include:

- skin—*Staphylococcus epidermidis*;
- nose—*Staphylococcus aureus*;
- mouth—*Streptococcus pyogenes*;
- intestines—*Clostridium tetani* (tetanus-causing bacteria), *Clostridium welchii* (gas gangrene-causing bacteria), and *E. coli.*

Interruption to transmission

Efforts to break the chain of infection must focus attention on the most vulnerable point in the chain (see Figure 1, p. 18). This will differ from case to case. In addition, consideration must be given to the route of infection. In particular, it is important to consider the following specific strategies:

- destroy the pathogenic agent by specific antibiotic therapy;
- control the reservoir of infection (for example, by isolating residents with highly contagious illnesses such as influenza);
- control the exit point (for example, by using sealed dressings or continence aids on infected residents, and staff covering their mouths when coughing or sneezing);
- control the transmission route by hand-washing, changing soiled working clothes, disinfection of equipment, and disinfection of excreta and other infected material);
- protect susceptible residents (for example, by controlling blood glucose levels of people with diabetes);
- increase residents' resistance by vaccination.[6]

Principles of infection prevention

The preferred method of preventing nosocomial infection is staff using barriers to interrupt the transmission of micro-organisms.

Historically, when an infectious disease was suspected or diagnosed, the patient was isolated. The current approach is to isolate all potential sources of infection, rather than the individual. This practice also offers protection from undiagnosed sources of infectious disease.

Recommended barrier or preventative aims include:

- documenting surveillance and treatment, and notifying any infections or infectious diseases;
- reducing person-to-person transmission opportunities;
- eliminating contamination by equipment;
- promoting cleaning and decontamination of the working environments;
- adopting standard and additional precautions policies, and practices; and
- promoting independence, good nutrition, and exercise for residents.

As well as creating barriers to the transmission of infection, it is important that staff members are consistent in their approach to infection prevention. A single action by one staff member, however perfect, is often fruitless. Success comes when the staff works as a team.

The most important barrier strategy is careful, correct, and regular hand-washing, because hand-washing reduces the transmission of micro-organisms.

Hand-washing

Hand-washing is the single most important practice to be mastered in infection control.

Hand-washing can be divided into three main types:[7]
1. routine, social, or mechanical hand-washing;
2. clinical hand-washing; and
3. surgical scrub.

Note: Alcoholic chlorhexidine can be used for hand-cleansing when hands are not visibly soiled and hand-washing facilities are not available.

The most commonly used type of hand-washing in residential facilities is *routine hand-washing*. Routine hand-washing assists with the removal and reduction of transient micro-organisms from the hands. Hands should be washed:

- whenever they are soiled;
- after toileting residents;
- before carrying out aseptic procedures;
- after carrying out a treatment and/or procedure on a resident;
- before and after performing dressings;
- after all resident contact (e.g., instilling eye drops);
- after handling contaminated equipment;
- after removing gloves; and
- before leaving, and returning to, the resident care area.

Staff members should remember the following points when washing their hands:

- any skin lesion that might compromise proper hand-washing must be reported to the unit manager;
- any skin breaks must be covered with a waterproof bandage or occlusive dressing;
- ornate rings, bracelets, and wrist watches should not be worn while giving direct care (because they prevent adequate hand-washing and can cause skin trauma to the resident); a plain wedding band is acceptable—only because few staff members are willing to remove their wedding rings to wash their hands;
- staff members should not use residents' washbasins unless there is no other basin available.
- the mechanical action of the hand-wash is more important than the product used; the washing action should be continuous for at least 20–30 seconds;
- soap and hand towels must be available at all washbasins; if soap dispensers are used they should be stabilised, easy to operate, and always contain lotion;
- bar soap can be used at hand basins provided the soap is rinsed under running water before use; however, care should be taken to safeguard mobile but disoriented residents from accidental ingestion of the bar soap;

- basic soap is adequate to remove transient micro-organisms in a routine hand-wash; however, an antiseptic agent should be used before performing invasive procedures;
- although it is an advantage for the taps on staff hand-basins to have elbow-operated arms or an electronic pump device, tap handles can be washed or turned off with paper towels to avoid recontaminating recently washed hands;
- the use of nail brushes is discouraged, because they cannot be adequately cleaned;
- linen towels must not be available at washbasins for communal use;
- the paper towel dispenser should be adjacent to the washbasin to avoid dropping water on the floor;
- a receptacle for used paper towels should be available close to the basin; the receptacle does not need a lid; and
- the use of hot-air dryers is discouraged because they are usually noisy and take too long to dry the hands (which encourages staff members to wipe their hands on clothing).

Standard precautions

Staff use of *standard precautions* (otherwise known as 'universal precautions' or 'body substance isolation') provides the basic level of infection control. Rather than waiting for a resident infection to be diagnosed before taking precautions to avoid spread, staff members who include these standard precautions in their resident care assume that *all* residents and staff members are potentially infected.

In residential facilities, infection is usually acquired:

- through an opening in the body via contaminated hands or materials;
- by blood-to-blood contact via broken skin or mucous membrane contact; or
- by inhaling airborne organisms.

Therefore the use of standard precautions is a recommended part of the care of all residents—regardless of the individual resident's perceived infectious status. Standard precautions are to be used whenever:

- body fluids are handled;
- contact is made with moist body surfaces; and
- contact is made with broken skin and mucous membranes.

Note: Staff who practise standard precautions routinely use barriers to prevent their own skin and mucous membranes coming into contact with blood or other body fluids.

These barriers include:

- effective hand washing;
- correct use of gloves, masks and protective eye wear;
- use of aseptic techniques;
- no-touch disposal of sharps; and
- careful disposal and handling of infectious waste.

Each staff member, according to the assessed risk in each situation, will determine the particular precautions required. However, people can 'carry' certain micro-organisms without showing obvious signs of illness. Consequently, when staff members adopt a standard precautions approach to all resident care, they protect residents, themselves, and other staff from contracting both diagnosed and undiagnosed infection.

In summary, implementation of standard precautions, or the use of barriers to avoid exposure to any body substances, prevents transmission of most infections by:

- assuming that all body fluids, tissues and moist surfaces are potentially infectious; and
- adopting barrier precautions in all situations where exposure to these substances is likely to occur.[8]

Additional precautions

Additional precautions can be used with standard precautions to form the second tier of infection control. Additional precautions are used in the care of residents known or suspected to be infected with, or colonised by, highly transmissible pathogens such as tuberculosis or VRE, which can cause infection by:

- airborne transmission;
- droplet transmission; or
- indirect or direct contact with dry skin or contaminated surfaces.

Because of the architectural design of the environment, if staff members use standard precautions there should rarely be a need to isolate a resident.

It can be difficult to establish and maintain additional precautions in some facilities. It might be more appropriate to transfer the resident to a hospital or facility where he or she can be treated safely without risk or threat to other residents and staff.

However, the additional precaution of segregating a resident from others is appropriate under the following circumstances if:

- the person's body substances cannot be contained (e.g., profuse and uncontrollable diarrhoea);

- the person has an undiagnosed productive cough (which might later be found to be due to an infectious condition).
- the person has influenza—because it is highly contagious;
- the person has a herpes zoster infection such as varicella (chickenpox) or shingles;
- the person has known or suspected active tuberculosis; or
- the person has an infectious disease and poor hygiene practices.

Resistant organisms[9]

MRSA

Multiple-resistant (or methicillin-resistant) *Staphylococcus aureus* (MRSA) has been the major agent of nosocomial cross-infection in Australian hospitals for more than 20 years. Although no more pathogenic than other strains of *Staphylococcus aureus*, the presence of MRSA in health-care institutions has become a problem because of:

- its ability to survive in a dry environment, making it easily transmitted via dry hands or fomites (inanimate objects);
- its ability to readily colonise humans without necessarily causing disease; and
- its resistance to most commonly used antibiotics.

The spectrum of disease caused by MRSA is broad—ranging from asymptomatic colonisation to deep abscesses and life-threatening septicaemia. Human reservoirs of MRSA include:

- people with MRSA colonisation of the nose, axilla, or groin;
- people with damaged skin; and
- people with active MRSA infection (for example, in a wound or sputum).

The most common mode of transmission of MRSA is by transient contamination of a staff member's hands—for example after contact with infected body fluids. Therefore, the possibility of transmitting the organism can be greatly reduced by staff members paying rigorous attention to hand-washing before and after contact with any person.

Although MRSA is such a major problem that complex control procedures and policies have been introduced in some health-care facilities, the correct focus of MRSA infection control is on improving poor standards of hygiene and infection-control practices. Routine screening of residents or staff is unnecessary. Infected residents should be managed according to standard precautions.

Occasional cases of MRSA infection are inevitable in facilities, given the prevalence of colonisation and the frequency of resident transfers between health-care facilities. Should an outbreak of nosocomial MRSA infection occur, staff members should investigate the chain of transmission and take the control steps necessary for any other nosocomial outbreak. In the process it might be found that many residents have undiagnosed colonisation with MRSA.

VRE[10]

Vancomycin-resistant enterococcus (VRE) emerged as a concern in acute-care facilities in 1994. At present there is no specific drug therapy available to combat VRE.

Various strains of *Enterococcus* are normal flora of the gastrointestinal tract. In addition, in up to 25 per cent of healthy individuals, this organism can also be found in such diverse locations as the oropharynx, vagina, urethra, and skin.

Enterococcal bacteria are most commonly spread from person-to-person by:

- direct contact;
- transient contamination of the hands of a staff member; and
- indirect contact with contaminated environmental surfaces.

Predisposing factors to VRE infection include:

- immunosuppression—because resistance is weakened;
- the use of broad-spectrum antibiotics; and
- a prolonged hospital stay (which increases the likelihood of exposure).

Chapter 2

Staff

Introduction

Health-care staff members have specific responsibilities when it comes to controlling infection in the workplace. As well as providing safe, informed care for residents, staff members have a responsibility to ensure they do not act as reservoirs of infection. In addition to having infection-control responsibilities in the course of their work, staff members are also exposed to specific infection-control risks. Infection control is often identified as a staff competency on position descriptions. In this chapter, both staff responsibilities and staff risks will be discussed.

Staff responsibilities

Professional care givers and support staff who work in residential-care facilities have personal infection-control responsibilities. As well as assessing the infection-control risk at every point of resident contact, staff members contribute to breaking the chain of infection by:

- maintaining a high standard of personal hygiene and grooming;
- monitoring their own health status; and
- maintaining recommended personal immunisation levels.

Staff hygiene and grooming

A high standard of personal hygiene and grooming is expected of those who work in the residential-care environment. Individual staff members must take responsibility for meeting the following hygiene and grooming standards.

Hands are the most likely contact point in the transmission of micro-organisms. Hands must be kept in a condition that optimises infection control. This involves:

- learning and practising good technique in hand-washing;
- keeping fingernails clean and short;
- using moisturisers to improve the condition of the skin;
- using waterproof protective dressings to cover open cuts and abrasions; and
- seeking prompt diagnosis of skin lesions (such as sores or rashes).

Daily showering is required, with additional washing of any part of the staff member's body that comes into unprotected contact with residents' blood or body fluids.

Hair must be clean and secured off the face for occupational health and safety and infection control. Some facilities require staff who work in food services wear to a cap to cover their hair, preventing micro-organisms falling from their hair into the food.

Jewellery worn on the hands or wrists must be removed when attending to residents. All rings, except for a plain wedding band, must be removed before hand-washing.

Clothing for work, whether uniform or street clothes, should be clean and changed each day to decrease the chance of cross-infection. Protective apparel is to be worn when necessary (see Chapter 4).

Unit managers must:

- set a good example by good personal hygiene practices;
- enforce standards of personal hygiene among the staff in their area; and
- communicate with management if any staff member in their area seems unable to meet the required standards of hygiene.

Managers must:

- inform staff of hygiene requirements during the recruitment process;
- provide staff with detailed instructions about hygiene requirements as part of the orientation process; and
- reinforce staff understanding of the importance of personal hygiene during regular infection-control education.

Staff health

Staff members who are at at risk of contracting or transmitting infection during their occupational activities owe it to themselves, their colleagues, and the residents in their care to monitor and maintain good personal health that will enable them to resist infection. Staff members' resistance to infection is likely to be highest if they:

- eat a well-balanced diet;
- obtain adequate rest, sleep, and exercise; and
- seek prompt diagnosis and treatment of any personal illness.

In addition, staff members must be alert for any symptoms that indicate that they might pose a significant risk of infecting others.

Early detection and reporting of staff infection plays an important role in breaking the chain of nosocomial infection. Staff members must contact their unit manager, prior to attending for work, if they are suffering from any of the following:

- fever;
- sore throat;
- productive cough;
- flu-like illness;

- acute skin eruption or infection;
- diarrhoea;
- conjunctivitis;
- wound discharge;
- jaundice;
- recent immunisation with a live virus vaccine such as oral poliomyelitis vaccine; or
- symptoms suggestive of scabies e.g. itching of skin folds.

The unit manager might suggest that the staff member remains away from work until cleared to return by a medical practitioner.

However staff members who have an established diagnosis of an infectious disease are not obliged to inform management—unless they might present an infectious risk to others. Management must maintain strict confidentiality regarding reports of staff illness.[1]

Staff immunisation[2]

Any health-care worker with frequent direct contact with residents will be exposed to a variety of serious infectious diseases that are preventable by immunisation. To avoid the possibility of acting as a reservoir of serious infection, all staff members are expected to:

- be aware of their personal infectious-diseases history (especially exposure to varicella, hepatitis, and AIDS) and their immunisation status against measles, mumps, poliomyelitis, rubella, tuberculosis and tetanus.
- be aware of, and keep records of, all immunisations;
- ensure that vaccinations and boosters are current.

Database

Health-care establishments should maintain a *database* or register that contains details about: (i) staff vaccination against preventable diseases; (ii) antibody and test results; (iii) a record of vaccinations to which the staff member consented or refused (including batch numbers and brand names of relevant vaccinations).

This register must be maintained by a designated staff member, updated regularly and kept in accordance with privacy and confidentiality legislation. The information should be accessible to authorised personnel if required.[3] This information can be difficult to acquire, and some staff members might not be willing to supply such information—especially if their general practitioner keeps such records for them. It might therefore be difficult to ascertain the vaccination status of staff against hepatitis B and influenza at any given time.

Staff members who received routine childhood immunisations can assume that they have completed courses of triple antigen vaccine (tetanus, diphtheria, and pertussis) and polio vaccine.

Booster doses

Booster doses are no longer recommended routinely for people who have had a full primary course of the three diphtheria-containing vaccines and at least two boosters. Immunity acquired following such a course is long-lasting.[4]

Polio boosters are given: (i) before starting school; and (ii) if the individual is at specific risk (e.g., staff members travelling to countries where poliomyelitis is endemic or staff members who are in contact with a case of poliomyelitis).[4]

Staff members who received a primary course of three doses of tetanus vaccine as adults should receive two booster doses at ten-year intervals. Immunity following complete vaccination is long-lasting. A booster dose is recommended at age 50, unless the person received a booster within ten years. Older adults who did not receive a booster at age 50 should receive a booster if more than ten years have elapsed since their last booster dose.[4]

Recommended immunisations

Recommended immunisations for health-care workers are as follows.

Rubella vaccine (single dose) is given to males and females whose antibodylevels indicate that they have never been infected with the virus. The rubella vaccine can be given combined with measles/mumps vaccine (MMR II) if there is no past history of these infections.

Hepatitis B vaccine is recommended for health-care workers who are frequently exposed to blood or body fluids in their work environment and/or staff members who are at occupational risk of needle-stick injury. Three doses of vaccine are given over 26 weeks, and the staff member's antibody status is assessed at least six weeks after the final dose. Evidence indicates that a completed primary course of hepatitis B vaccination provides long-lasting protection in immuno-competent individuals, and booster doses are therfore not recommended.[4] However, booster doses are recommended for immuno-suppressed individuals, for people with HIV infection, and for those with renal failure. [4]

Tuberculosis vaccination (BCG) can be given to staff members who are considered to be at risk of acquiring tuberculosis (TB) and who have a negative Mantoux skin test. A trained person injects a small quantity of tuberculin under the skin to perform a Mantoux skin test. The area is checked for a positive reaction three days later. The use of BCG vaccine in occupational settings is debatable, because a positive Mantoux skin test can be the result of a previous BCG or exposure to a person with TB.

Influenza vaccine is recommended annually for: (i) all adults more than 65 years of age; (ii) all Aboriginal and Torres Strait Islander peoples older than 50 years; (iii) people with a chronic illness; and (iv) residents of nursing homes and other long-stay facilities. Staff working with these individuals should also consider having the influenza vaccination.[4]

A doctor or accredited immunisation nurse should take responsibility for staff immunisation processes.

Transport, storage, and handling of vaccines

Vaccines should be transported in an insulated container with approved temperature-monitoring processes. They should not be frozen or come in direct contact with ice packs.

If a vaccine has been exposed to temperatures lower than 2–8 degrees Celsius they might be no longer viable. Check the expiry date on the vial or container before storage, and rotate stock so that the shortest 'in date' vaccines are used first.

Situations of high infection risk

Staff members who are exposed to situations of high infection risk—such as needle-stick injury, or exposure to body substances—require special precautions.

When a staff member suffers a significant exposure to a body substance, careful and systematic followup by a medical practitioner or prescribed person (a person trained in counselling and followup) is recommended.

A significant exposure is one in which body substances are injected into the staff member:

- by a used needle (needle-stick injury);
- in any puncture wound;
- as a result of laceration by a contaminated sharp instrument; or
- as a result of the staff member's mucous membranes (particularly those in the eye or mouth) come into contact with another person's blood.

Razor blades, used scalpels and scissors can be a potential source of staff exposure to residents' body fluids.

A staff member is also at risk if bitten by a resident, although the resident is also at significant risk (due to exposure to the staff member's blood).

The risk of transmission of serious viral illnesses such as the human immune-deficiency virus (HIV) from accidental needle stick injury is very low. This depends on such factors as:

- the concentration of the virus in the contaminating body fluid;
- the volume of body fluid injected; and
- whether the needle was hollow or solid.

The same treatment applies whether the exposed person is a staff member, resident, or visitor.

First aid

Immediately after the exposure or injury:

- wash the affected area thoroughly;
- if there is a wound, do not encourage bleeding and do not further traumatise the area;
- if a mucous membrane is involved, wash or irrigate it with warm water or saline.

Assessing the injury or exposure[6]

1. Immediate notification

The injured or exposed staff member must immediately inform the unit manager. As soon as possible after first aid, the staff member must complete an incident form—recording the following information:

- type of exposure (blood splash, needle-stick, laceration from a contaminated sharp, human bite, contact with intact or non intact skin);
- details of the body site of the exposure;
- a description of events resulting in exposure; and
- the precautions that were taken (if any); and
- whether first aid was given.

The incident report must be completed whether or not the exposure is considered significant. The report should be forwarded promptly to the director of nursing or manager of the facility.

2. Referral

The unit manager must refer the staff member promptly to a medical practitioner (designated by the facility), a prescribed person, or the staff member's own general practitioner.

3. Role of practitioner

The medical practitioner or prescribed person must determine the significance of the exposure and decide on recommended action.

4. Role of management

Management is obliged to:

- maintain strict confidentiality regarding follow up and pathology results;
- properly assess the circumstances surrounding the incident;
- address any problems found (in order to prevent a recurrence of the incident); and
- include the report of the incident in quality-improvement activities.

If the exposure is significant and the disease status of the source person (e.g. the resident whose blood was on the needle) is unknown, consideration should be given to requesting tests for HIV, hepatitis B, and hepatitis C from the source person. Such tests will be allowed only after gaining the informed consent of the source person or his or her guardian.

Action following the assessment of the injury or exposure

1. Tetanus

Tetanus toxoid immunisation should be considered if the sharp item involved in the exposure has been in contact with other contaminated material (such as garbage or garden soil).

2. Hepatitis B

Appropriate action in the case of exposure to hepatitis B depends on the immunisation status of the exposed person. It might be desirable to administer immunoglobulin soon after the event if the exposed person has not had the condition or has not been immunised against it.

3. HIV

Antiviral chemoprophylaxis might be offered by a medical practitioner to a staff member who has been exposed to a source of HIV. Chemoprophylaxis has not proven successful in all cases of significant exposure to HIV and can produce undesirable side-effects.

Following exposure to HIV, the affected person should be encouraged to:

- report any signs or symptoms that might indicate acute HIV seroconversion (such as a transient rash or fever occurring within three months of the exposure);
- return to the doctor or counsellor for advice or discussion if concerned; and
- return to the doctor for reassessment at specific, regular intervals over the following year.

Until follow-up blood tests are complete, health-care workers exposed to HIV and/or hepatitis B should practise safe sex and refrain from donating blood.

To ensure confidentiality, any request slips and specimens tested can be coded. Results of tests are usually available within 24-hours after the blood is taken.

4. Counselling

There is a wide range of possible psychological reactions to a significant exposure to blood or other body fluids. Any person (staff, resident or visitor) who needs an HIV test as a result of such an incident should be offered qualified counselling before and after the test.

Personnel policies for HIV, hepatitis B, and hepatitis C infection

Staff members who have been infected with HIV, hepatitis B, or hepatitis C (or think they might have been):

- are not obliged to inform their employer of their condition;
- have a duty to act responsibly towards their fellow workers by: (i) obtaining medical assistance to monitor their own health; (ii) being vigilant in preventing their blood and body fluids from coming into contact with other people; (iii) acknowledging that it is illegal to put another person at risk knowingly, willingly, and recklessly.

The effects of bloodborne illnesses are such that affected staff members might require intermittent sick leave. As with any other employee illness, employers have a responsibility to accommodate the legitimate leave requirements of staff with bloodborne diseases.

Tuberculosis screening for health-care workers[5]

Guidelines for health-care workers are available from health departments in all states. These advise that staff who work in facilities such as private hospitals, country hospitals, and residential facilities are at low risk of becoming infected with TB from their residents and clients.

If a resident is discovered to have active TB, staff members at high risk of exposure will be screened by the public health unit of their state health department. They might require chest X-ray or preventative therapy, especially after exposure to residents with multi-resistant tuberculosis organisms.

Staff members who have had a successful BCG vaccination will usually be protected against TB. Evidence of successful immunisation is the characteristic scar (usually on the upper arm or outside of the thigh). Revaccination with BCG is unlikely, except in special circumstances. Staff screened for TB will be given a written record of the outcome to keep.

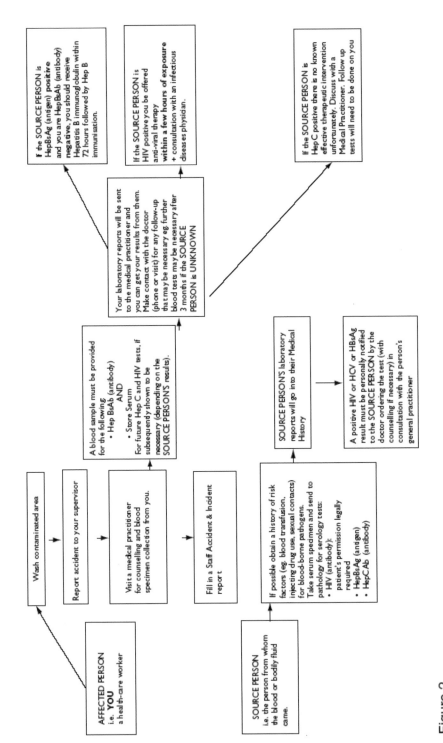

Figure 2
What to do if you have a needle stick or blood splash accident.

Chapter 3

Residents

Introduction

This chapter begins by presenting general preventative strategies, and concludes with information about specific infectious agents commonly encountered in aged-care facilities. The information in this section offers staff members an opportunity to:

- increase their risk-assessment skills;
- plan appropriate infection-control interventions; and
- provide optimum resident care.

Factors predisposing residents to infection

In order to resist infection, an individual requires a healthy and efficient immune system. The ability to produce a healthy immune response to the threat of infection at any body site is dependent on various factors, including:

- intact skin and mucous membranes (the primary barrier to the entry of micro-organisms);
- adequate production of mature, infection-fighting white blood cells;
- efficient circulation (including heart and vascular system) to increase the blood flow and white blood cell supply to any area of inflammation or infection;
- adequate management of physical, mental, and emotional stress; and
- adequate diet, rest, and sleep.

As individuals age, their immune systems, like all other body systems, become less efficient. For this reason, older residents will have reduced defence mechanisms and be at risk of infection.

Certain factors predispose any resident to infection. When assessing a resident's infection risk, staff members need to consider the following risk factors:

- general susceptibility;
- local susceptibility; and
- environmental factors.

1. General susceptibility

General susceptibility includes:

- poor hygiene, which increases the number and types of microorganisms on the resident's skin;
- poor nutritional status, which reduces the resident's resistance to infection;

- obesity, which inhibits the resident's circulation and ability to self-care;
- mental disturbance, which increases the resident's feelings of stress and which interferes with the resident's ability to self-care;
- prolonged time spent in hospital prior to admission to the facility, which increases the resident's exposure to a range of micro-organisms;
- treatment with cytotoxic drugs, radiotherapy or cortisone and related drugs, which reduces the resident's resistance to infection; and
- underlying diseases such as diabetes, vascular disease or chronic leukaemia, which can interfere with circulation and inhibit the supply of mature white blood cells.

2. Local susceptibility

Local susceptibility factors include:

- dehydration, which can lead to drying and cracking of skin and mucous membrane;
- immobility (e.g., following stroke or other brain injury), which can predispose the resident to poor circulation and inhibiting the ability to self-care;
- invasive procedures, such as urinary catheterisation;
- the presence of a foreign body in the body tissue;
- infections elsewhere in the body, which can lower the resident's resistance; and
- low resistance to bacterial colonisation of some body tissues (such as the inner part of the eye, brain, joints, and urinary tract), which can make residents susceptible to infection at these sites by opportunistic organisms.

3. Environmental factors

Environmental factors include:

- carers with little or no knowledge of infection control who inadvertently put the resident at risk of cross infection; and
- unsuitable design of the facility (e.g., limited access to toilets, inaccessible hand-basins or lack of a pan sanitiser), which can increase the risk of cross infection.

General precautions to protect residents

As discussed earlier, standard precautions assume that the body substances of *all* residents and staff are potentially infectious—rather than requiring a specific diagnosis of infection before infection-control precautions are taken.

If staff and management understand what predisposes residents to infection, and if they use appropriate precautions, it is possible to develop strategies that augment residents' immune functioning. Staff in each facility will be able to add to the following basic list of suggested strategies:

- providing emotional support to a newly admitted resident;
- training staff to recognise depressed or anxious residents (and provide appropriate therapeutic responses);
- boosting residents' self-esteem (for example, by offering music, validation, and reminiscence therapies);
- promoting residents' independence and self-caring abilities;
- providing mobilisation and exercise programs;
- scheduling regular physical assessment of residents to identify underlying disease;
- rotating menus and providing residents with a choice of meals;
- introducing strategies to enhance residents' night sleep;
- offering additional fluids in warm weather;
- training staff in infection control and wound care;
- ensuring residents have skin-moisturising products;
- encouraging staff members to wash their hands; and
- managing urinary incontinence without catheterisation (if possible).

Specific precautions to protect residents

Specific strategies can be used to combat the infection-control risks posed by:

- urinary catheterisation;
- enteral feeding;
- intravenous therapy;
- residents with tuberculosis;
- residents with vancomycin-resistant enterococcus (VRE); and
- an outbreak of scabies.

Each of these is discussed in the following pages.

Note: For further information on urinary catheterisation and enteral feeding, refer to Chapter 4, 'Infection Control Procedures and Practices'.

Urinary catheterisation

The widespread use of urinary catheterisation to manage incontinence should be discouraged because the presence of an indwelling urinary catheter almost always increases the number of micro-organisms in the urine. Antibiotic therapy for residents with urinary catheters will not stop infections occurring because the foreign body of the catheter makes the resident locally susceptible.

Careful infection-control management of the catheter will minimise the infection risk to the resident. Because the outside of the catheter cannot be kept sterile, the single most important aspect of catheter care is that the drainage system should remain closed. It is therefore vital to ensure that the interior of the catheter, the attached drainage bag, and the bladder lumen have no communication with the outside environment, and that the system is not breached (except for good reason such as changing the bag). If a breach is necessary, strict aseptic technique must be used.

All catheterised residents must be monitored for infection. Staff should document the following:

- fever;
- foul-smelling urine;
- suprapubic pain or tenderness; and
- behaviour changes (such as restlessness, confusion, or drowsiness).

Antibiotics might be appropriate at the time of insertion and removal of the catheter (when the risk of infection is greatest). A single dose of broad spectrum antibiotic should be considered for:

- residents whose immune defences are seriously compromised (e.g., residents on immunosuppressive medication such as prednisolone or cytotoxic medication);
- residents showing signs of serious infection (e.g., fever, lower abdominal pain).

Antibiotics should be prescribed according to recommended guidelines based on the result of the urine culture and sensitivity.

Enteral feeding

The practice of enteral feeding is widespread in aged-care facilities because it offers an acceptable alternative to the discomfort of nasogastric feeding for residents who are unable to swallow nutrients—for example, following a cerebrovascular accident (CVA).

Particular care must be paid to infection control when storing or handling the feeding formula and equipment because:

- the feed is often milk-based and therefore provides an environment in which micro-organisms can readily multiply;
- the gastrostomy is an unnatural opening into a body cavity, thus bypassing the normal mechanisms that protect against the invasion of bacteria; and
- residents who need enteral feeding are often frail and dependent, and are therefore more likely to be susceptible to infection.

Intravenous (IV) therapy

The principles of asepsis must be maintained during insertion and removal of the cannula and when IV therapy is in progress. These include:

- clinical hand-washing at the time of insertion and removal of the cannula;
- correct skin preparation before insertion;
- maintaining a sterile field during insertion;
- placing a sterile dressing over the insertion site after the procedure;
- maintaining a patent line to prevent phlebitis; and
- resiting the cannula and lines every 48–72 hours

With respect to the last point, the date when each cannula was inserted should be recorded in the resident's medical history (and on the dressing over the IV site).

Tuberculosis[1]

Tuberculosis (TB) is increasing in the general population after a period of decline. It is therefore possible that staff members will care for a resident with active pulmonary TB at some time. The term 'active TB' means there is evidence of the organism in the infected person's sputum.

If a resident is found to have a positive TB sputum culture, management will put into place certain precautions (in consultation with the resident's medical officer). The resident will be isolated in a single room with:

- negative air pressure or externally exhausted air;
- separate air conditioning; and
- ensuite facilities.

If ensuite facilities are not available, the resident should be allocated a room as close as possible to a shower and toilet dedicated to that resident's use alone. If isolation conditions are unsatisfactory, consideration should be given to transferring the resident temporarily to a hospital with proper isolation facilities.

Other infection-control measures for TB include:

- *Masks:* Staff members having close or prolonged contact with any resident with active TB should wear high-efficiency filter masks. In addition, while the resident is considered infectious, masks must be worn by any staff members in direct contact with the resident (including cleaning staff), by the infectious resident (when outside the isolation area), and by visitors (when visiting the isolated person).
- *Gowns:* Gowns must be worn by staff members who are providing direct resident care and by visitors when visiting the isolated person. However, gowns must be removed before leaving the isolation area.
- *Crockery and cutlery:* If kitchen practices follow recommended guidelines, no additional precautions are required.[2,3]
- *Disposal of body fluids:* Disposal of body fluids (such as infected sputum from a person with pulmonary TB, or urine from a person with renal TB) must comply with standard guidelines and additional precautions guidelines.

Note: Staff members whose own immunity is compromised by chronic illness should not care for residents with active TB.

Vancomycin-resistant enterococcus[4]

As previously discussed, enterococcal varieties of bacteria are normal flora in a number of body sites, including the gastrointestinal tract. However, infection with vancomycin-resistant enterococcus (VRE) is of concern because there is, at present, no effective antibiotic therapy.

VRE is spread by person-to-person contact. A recently admitted resident, or a resident returning from a stay in a major hospital, might be colonised with VRE.

Because of the risk to other residents, the following precautions must be observed:

- staff must use standard and additional precautions when caring for a resident with VRE infection;

- if a single room is not available in the facility, the affected resident must share a room only with residents who are likely to have strong and intact immune defences;
- when the resident is discharged or transferred, equipment in the resident's room should be disinfected with sodium hypochlorite 500 ppm, after thorough washing with hot soapy water;
- communally used equipment (such as lifting straps) must be disinfected after use on an infected resident;
- thorough washing with hot soapy water must be followed by a wipe-down with hypochlorite 500 ppm; and
- all staff, and visitors to the infected resident, must be educated about the prevention of VRE transmission;

No special precautions are needed for dishes, glasses, cups, or eating utensils. The hot water and detergents used in institutional dishwashers are sufficient to decontaminate these items. Special handling of contaminated waste is not required unless authorities require supervised landfill disposal. For linen handling, follow the general guidelines in Chapter 5.

If a resident does not need assistance with activities of daily living and is continent, the risk of transmission to others is lower. Residents who are colonised or infected with multiresistant bacteria need not be restricted to their rooms. However, before using communal areas, they should change into clean clothing and be encouraged or assisted to wash their hands.

Infected residents who are incontinent of faeces must be confined to their rooms while the incontinence persists.

Note: If more detailed guidance is required, staff and management are advised to obtain the latest guidelines from state health authorities, such as the Victorian Department of Human Services' *Infection Control Guidelines for the Management of Patients with Methicillin Resistant Staphylococcus Aureus (MRSA) and Vancomycin Resistant Enterococci (VRE) in Long Term Care Facilities (LTCF)*.

Scabies infestation

On admission to the facility, residents should be visually screened for abnormalities of the skin—especially rashes, track marks, or burrows in the finger-web areas. Any suspect lesions should be scraped and a specimen sent to the laboratory for identification.

If a resident is confirmed as having scabies staff who have been in contact with the person, and residents who share the same bedroom, must be checked for visible signs of scabies infestation.

Until the infestation has been treated (see Chapter 7), the affected resident must be isolated and staff attending to the resident must take the special precautions of wearing gloves and gown (single use).

At the same time as the skin is being treated, bed linen and clothing should be thoroughly laundered, and rooms should be thoroughly cleaned. Residents must never share shower caps or clothing.

To avoid infecting others it might be necessary to segregate the infested person from others until the treatment is complete.

If the infestation recurs despite adequate treatment, environmental sampling of bedside dust should be undertaken, and rooms can be carefully sprayed with a domestic insecticide.

Chapter 4

Infection Control Procedures

and Practices

Introduction

In residential aged care, the resident is the centre of all care activities. However, in terms of infection control, three distinct components in the chain of infection can be identified:

- the actions of the staff;
- management of equipment; and
- procedures required by the residents.

In practice, infection control activity cannot be easily divided, because each component forms a part of the others. However, by observing infection-control principles in all aspects of resident care, including specific procedures, staff can ensure that the chain of infection is broken.

1. Staff-centred procedures

Hand-washing

As previously noted, the most important infection-control procedure is staff members washing their hands. Posters should be placed above hand basins. These should: (i) state when hands should be washed; and (ii) demonstrate how they should be washed.

Hand washing must be thorough and systematic, and should be carried out:

- before all aseptic procedures;
- after attending to residents;
- before and after staff breaks;
- after disposing of potentially infected materials; and
- whenever hands are inadvertently contaminated.

Procedure for routine hand-washing[1]

1. Start by wetting the hands under warm, running water. Using the volume of cleansing lotion obtained from one depression of the dispenser pump, begin to lather the hands. From this point a set routine is needed to ensure that the solution contacts all surfaces.

2. Move from the palms to the side surfaces of the thumbs, and from the right hand to the left. Then entwine the fingers and work them back and forth along the full length of the fingers.

3. Next, wash the back of the right hand and make a few twists around the wrist. Wash the backs of the fingers and the thumb. Then move to the finger-webs with intertwined fingers.

4. Repeat this procedure on the back of the left hand.

5. Finally, work the tips of the fingers and thumbs into the palm of the each hand, making sure that the solution finds its way behind and under the nails.

6. Now rinse. This is important. If the cleanser is not rinsed off carefully, the skin will become dry. Slant the hands down so that the water drains from the fingers into the sink.

7. Turn the taps off with the elbows, or holding a paper towel in the hand, to ensure that hands are not recontaminated.

8. Dry hands thoroughly. Cultures taken from wet hands provide ample evidence that bacteria multiply more rapidly under these conditions than on dry skin.

As discussed in Chapter 1, the 20–30-second duration of a routine hand-wash provides enough time for the solution to remove transient organisms.

Procedure for clinical hand-washing[2]

A clinical hand-wash is required before commencing an aseptic technique—such as a wound dressing or catheterisation.

During a clinical hand-wash, hands and forearms are washed with antibacterial solution for one minute, or according to the recommendation of the manufacturer of the solution. The hands are then rinsed, with the flow of water directed from the hands to elbows.

Note: Videos and posters depicting correct hand-washing procedures are available from some pharmaceutical suppliers.

Protective clothing[3]

Gloves

Disposable gloves should be worn to prevent soiling the hands with blood or other body substances—for example, when handling potentially contaminated equipment (such as urinary drainage bags). Disposable gloves should be strategically placed at central locations for easy access when urgently required. The practice of routinely wearing gloves or carrying them in pockets should be discouraged. Although the gloves might protect the wearer's skin, they also provide an ideal medium for transporting organisms.

Sterile gloves should be worn for procedures where strict asepsis is required—for example, insertion of indwelling urinary catheters.

Gloves are a layer of protection, in addition to intact skin. However, the need to wear gloves varies with the skill of the staff member and the degree of cooperation of the resident. Some staff members might experience a loss of dexterity when wearing gloves.

Regardless of staff preferences, the following guidelines should be considered:

- wearing gloves does not eliminate the need to wash hands;
- gloves are not required for contact with intact skin and mucous membranes;
- gloves must be worn if a staff member has skin breaches on his or her hands;
- gloves are not necessary for removing bedpans and urinals from continent residents, provided the equipment was sited correctly;
- when changing the beds of incontinent residents a 'no-touch' technique should be used, rather than the routine use of gloves; however, if a resident is uncooperative and unpredictable, gloves should be worn;
- gloves must never be washed and then worn when attending to another resident; washing causes flaws in the gloves and this can allow permeation of fluid and organisms;
- gloves must be removed after each interaction with a resident, and the hands washed after the gloves have been removed; and
- unless they are heavily contaminated, gloves can be disposed of into general waste containers; if heavily contaminated, they should be disposed of into yellow infectious or clinical waste bags.

Gowns and plastic aprons

Staff clothing is a potential means of transmission of respiratory organisms, skin infections, and infestations (such as scabies). Wearing a gown or plastic apron over staff clothing can prevent contaminating clothing when handling contaminated equipment and biological substances. However, the following points should be observed.

- Cotton gowns or disposable plastic aprons are required only during procedures in which clothing is likely to be contaminated by body substances—for example, bowel washouts, enemas, or if the resident has a major skin break.
- It is better to wear a plastic apron than a cloth gown because soiling on a gown can soak through the cloth onto the wearer's clothing. Plastic aprons are also cheaper than gowns and offer more protection from splashes and body fluids.
- When wearing a gown, ensure that the top and waist ties are secure.
- The gown must be removed for washing after completing the procedure and must not be worn when attending to the next resident because this increases the risk of cross infection.
- Gowns must not be worn outside the resident care area.
- Wearing multi-use aprons should be discouraged because they are rarely cleaned and therefore pose an infection risk.

Masks

Masks must be worn for any procedure that could result in the face or mouth coming into contact with body fluids—for example, airborne droplets from a resident with an uncontrollable, productive cough.

Facemasks inhibit the dispersal of organisms, but they do not completely prevent droplet infection. Therefore coughing or conversation should be kept to a minimum during a procedure.

The effectiveness of masks is short-lived, but using a mask does provide some protection. In the absence of a mask, keeping the mouth shut will reduce the risk of infection.

Hands should be washed after putting on a mask. Masks must be:

- fluid-repellent; paper masks are of little use;
- worn for aseptic procedures;
- able to fit the face and cover the nose and the mouth untouched while in position on the face;
- used only once and never placed in pockets after use;
- removed by handling the tapes only;
- disposed of immediately after removal; and
- never left hanging around the neck.

Protective eye wear

The eye is exposed to organisms via the airborne route, and infection can therefore occur during certain procedures. Devices such as goggles, glasses, or visors are recommended for use if any contact with body fluids is likely. Protective eye wear must be worn if there is a possibility that infected material could be sprayed (for example, when cleaning bedpans or wound forceps).

Eye protection:

- should be available in both clean and dirty utility rooms; and
- must be worn when cleaning any equipment contaminated with body fluids.

Protective eyewear:

- must be washed with detergent to remove contaminating material; and
- must be frequently cleaned.

It should be noted that contact lenses will not protect eyes.

2. Equipment-oriented procedures

Managing sharps[4]

Safe disposal of single-use, sharp articles and instruments (such as needles and scalpel blades) is necessary to prevent injury and possible transmission of disease. Sharps must be disposed of into a stable, rigid-walled container.

The following procedures should be observed.

- It is preferable to take the rigid-walled sharps container to the site of the procedure before commencing the procedure.
- The person who generates a sharp for disposal should be the person who places the sharp into an appropriate container.
- Sharp objects must never be passed directly between people.
- Distractions should be avoided when sharps are being handled.
- Recapping needles (reinserting into their original sheath) is unacceptable practice.
- Needles and syringes must not be separated by hand before disposal. The needle should be left on the syringe for disposal. (De-notching is discouraged, but is practised in some facilities.)
- Do not attempt to break or bend needles by hand.
- Butterfly needles must always be handled by their wings to prevent the needle flicking back and injuring the user.
- Dispose of disposable razors and safety razor blades into a sharps container.
- Sharps containers must comply with Australian Standards AS 4261 and AS 4031.
- To prevent overfilling, sharps containers must be sealed and changed when the specified level is reached. Never shake the container to lower the level.
- Residents or visitors should not have access to sharps containers.
- Full sharps containers must be incinerated, or treated according to the supplier's recommendations.
- Full sharps containers must be secured in a clean environment before collection. In country areas this might be a designated refrigerated area.

Managing specimens

Specimen collection is a potentially hazardous procedure for staff because of the possible contact with contaminated or infected body fluids. The following points should be observed for maximum protection.

- Containers should be labelled before taking a specimen.
- The container must be sealed immediately after collecting a specimen.
- Specimens do not require flagging (that is, identified as being from a known infectious person). If standard precautions are used, *every* specimen is regarded as potentially infectious.
- Specimen containers must be safely sealed in a labelled plastic bag for transporting to the laboratory.
- The request slip must remain separate from the specimen to prevent its becoming contaminated.
- Containers soiled on the outside with body fluids should be decontaminated with a chlorine compound (e.g., sodium hypochlorite or bleach).
- Specimens for microscopy and culture should be forwarded to the laboratory as soon as they are obtained.
- If there is a delay before transporting, the specimens should be stored in a designated area of the refrigerator used for medications, not a food refrigerator.
- Specimens should not be kept in offices.
- Unwanted specimens should be disposed of through the sewerage system.

Managing spills of biological material[5]

Under standard precautions *all* body fluids are regarded as potentially infectious. Spills of urine or blood must be therefore cleaned up with extreme care.

The first step is to stop and assess the volume of the spill and the nature of material to be removed. Using the cleaning approach that offers least risk of contamination, proceed in the following way:

1. Once the spill has been assessed, gather the necessary equipment. This includes:
   - disposable gloves;
   - absorbent paper towels;
   - plastic bag; and
   - forceps for picking up any sharps.
2. Put the gloves on.
3. Using gloved hands, cover the material with absorbent paper towel to contain the spill.
4. Gather up the contaminated material, and dispose of it into an 'infectious waste' bag.
5. Use forceps to pick up any sharps or broken glass and dispose of these appropriately.
6. Clean the area with hot water and detergent.

7. Sodium hypochlorite can be used if it is thought that there is a risk of exposure to the staff member, or if the spilled material is known to be infectious. It should be diluted to 500 ppm available chlorine for vancomycin-resistant enterococcus, 1000 ppm available chlorine for viral disinfection, or 10,000 ppm for blood spills.

8. Remove gloves and dispose of them into an 'infectious waste' bag.

If a spill occurs on carpet or soft furnishings chlorine might discolour the surface. Detergent can therefore be used, but the area should be cleaned and dried properly. A mop and bucket might be appropriate for a spill on a hard floor.

3. Resident-centred procedures

Enteral feeding

Procedure

After use, feeding containers must be rinsed in cold water to prevent the feed adhering to the container. The rinsed container should then be washed in detergent and water and stored clean and dry, ready for reuse by the same resident.

Giving sets and containers

The maximum life of a giving set is 3–7 days (or according to the manufacturer's recommendation). However, for optimum infection control, giving sets that are used continuously should be changed every 48-hours, and giving sets that are used intermittently should be changed every seven days—provided there are no signs or symptoms of infection and provided that the equipment is cleaned and stored correctly.

If syringe bolus feeding is practised, the syringe and plunger must be cleaned in hot soapy water after each use and stored clean and dry, ready for re-use by the same resident.

Feeds

Opened containers of unused formula must be dated and stored in the refrigerator in rust-proof containers and discarded after 24 hours. In hot weather, feeding regimens should be planned so that containers have only small volumes of feed. Large volumes of feed at room temperature will promote the growth of organisms.

Care of the gastrostomy tube

- Inspect the surrounding skin for redness, tenderness, swelling, irritation, purulent drainage, or gastric leakage.
- Cleanse the skin with soapy water, using a circular movement outwards from the stoma.
- Clean under the skin disc, and then dry the area thoroughly.
- Do not place dressings between the skin disc and the skin because this can encourage growth of organisms.
- Document observations made at the time of the procedure (for example, inflammation at the site).

Urinary catheters

Indwelling urinary catheters[6]

- Indwelling catheters must be inserted under sterile conditions using sterile, gloved hands and a 'no-touch' technique.
- Use only sterile water to inflate the balloon.
- Maintain a clean technique when emptying drainage bags.
- Care must be taken to avoid a kink in the tubing.
- The catheter bag must be kept below the bladder level.
- Bags must not touch, or be placed on the floor.
- Single-use bags must be changed when full. Bags that can be emptied should be changed weekly.
- The resident's personal hygiene must be maintained.
- Washing the genital area twice a day with soap and water will usually prevent contamination by micro-organisms.
- Where the catheter and urethra meet, keep the area clean and dry. Catheter dressings are not recommended.
- The application of antiseptics to the outside of the catheter is of little or no use.
- Immobilise the catheter to prevent micro-organisms being carried into the urethra on the surface of a moving catheter.
- The catheter and tubing should be led over the thigh, not under it, to minimise contamination of the outside of the catheter. Always attach the catheter or tubing to the resident, not to clothing and never to the bedclothes.
- Collect urine specimens for culture by inserting a needle in the rubber port of the tubing after swabbing the port with alcohol, rather than by disconnecting the catheter from the tubing.

- If it is necessary to close off the catheter, use an external clamp (rather than disconnecting the tubing and closing the catheter off with a spigot).
- Choose the smallest size of catheter possible (but not too small or it might buckle in the urethra during insertion).
- Leakage around a catheter indicates either a blocked catheter or bladder spasm. Changing the catheter for a bigger one will not alleviate the spasm.
- If leg bags are used, the overnight bag should be connected to the leg bag, so the point of connection is furthest from the bladder.
- Catheters and drainage bags must be used according to the manufacturer's guidelines. Cleaning and reusing drainage bags is *not* recommended.
- Bladder washouts should not be performed unless ordered by a medical practitioner.
- Latex catheters should not be considered for long-term use.
- Long-term catheters are available and can be used for up to 12 weeks. The date of insertion must be recorded in the resident's notes.

Condom drainage

A condom must be changed daily, with careful attention to washing and drying the penis. The resident's foreskin must be retracted during the cleaning process and then returned to its original position. Creams should not be applied because they can cause irritation and inflammation.

Chapter 5

Environment

Introduction

The residents' environment is larger than the area of the facility. The human environment of staff, residents' families, and social contacts extend the residents' world well beyond the walls of the facility and into the general community.

Although this broad understanding of 'environment' should be kept in mind when considering the chain of infection, for the purposes of this chapter the infection-control environment is limited to:

- the preparation and maintenance of resident care equipment;
- the type of supplies and equipment that staff members use in resident care;
- the effectiveness of environmental services (including the infection-control integrity of the facility's laundry and food services, and the facility's cleanliness); and
- the way in which pest infestation and waste disposal is managed.

When planning for and purchasing equipment, consideration should be given to infection control, occupational health and safety, and the cleaning, storage, maintenance and disposal of each piece of equipment.

Decontamination of resident equipment[1]

'Decontamination' is a general term for all methods of cleaning, disinfection, or sterilisation that are undertaken to remove microbial contaminants from equipment. The degree of decontamination required is determined by the risk of infection posed by the use of the particular instrument or piece of equipment.

Cleaning, disinfection, and sterilisation

Equipment used in resident care can be categorised according to the need for:

- cleaning (removal of bioburden from surfaces);
- disinfection (killing or removing most micro-organisms, with the exception of bacterial spores); or
- sterilisation (killing and removing all micro-organisms including bacterial spores).

In practice, instruments and equipment are often processed unnecessarily. Unnecessary sterilisation is costly in terms of processing materials and staff time (see Table 5.1, page 54).

Table 5.1: Levels of equipment processing[2]

1. Critical level of risk

Item application	Entry or penetration into sterile rissues, cavity, or blood stream
Decontamination process	Sterilisation by steam under pressure (autoclaving)
Storage after processing	Sterility must be maintained; packaged items must be allowed to dry before removal from the steriliser; the integrity of the wrap must be maintained
Example of item	Instruments used during podiatry procedures

2. Semi-critical level of risk

Item application	Contact with intact mucosa (or non-intact skin)
Decontamination process	Steam sterilisation is preferred
Storage after processing	Store to protect from environmental contamination
Example of item	Sigmoidoscope or vaginal speculum

3. Non-critical level of risk

Item application	Contact with intact skin
Decontamination process	Clean as necessary with detergent, then disinfect with 70% alcohol or other disinfectant as required
Storage after processing	Store in a clean dry place
Example of item	Stethescopes or blood pressure cuffs

If equipment that requires sterilisation is processed on site, compliance with the Australian/New Zealand Code of Practice AS/NZS 4187: 2003 involves careful documentation.[3] In the end it might be cost-effective to have any necessary processing done by an external agency (for example, a local hospital or medical centre).

Instruments used by external service providers (such as doctors and podiatrists) must be cleaned, sterilised, packaged, stored, and transported in compliance with Australian/New Zealand Standard AS/NZS 4187: 2003.

If only forceps and scissors are to be processed, the use of disposable dressing packs and single-use instruments (such as sterile blades or stitch cutters) might be a less expensive and more convenient option for a residential facility. In this way, although some equipment will still require decontamination, neither a steriliser (with its maintenance requirements) nor a contract (with an external facility) will be required.

The information in this chapter will help facility management and staff to identify which items must be disinfected, and which need to be sterilised.[4]

Cleaning

Physical cleaning must be performed before disinfection or sterilisation to increase the effectiveness of the process. After cleaning:

- there are fewer micro-organisms to kill;
- all surfaces become fully exposed;
- inactivating substances are removed; and
- the working life of the item is prolonged.

The mechanical action of cleaning is as important as the product used. The suggested process is as follows:

1. Dismantle or open items, as appropriate.

2. Rinse, clean and flush the item in running water at a temperature of 15–30°C to remove any visible blood or body substances. Blood or any other protein-based substance will coagulate and become firmly fixed to an item at higher temperatures, enabling micro-organisms to survive the sterilisation process.

3. Wash the equipment in warm water (45°C) and detergent at the recommended concentration.

4. Hold the item low in the sink to limit aerosol spray during washing.

5. Wash all surfaces, including any lumens or inner surfaces.

6. Rinse in warm to hot running water.

7. Dry the instruments.

8. Check the instruments for cleanliness.

Care must be taken to prevent penetration of the skin or splashing mucous membranes during the cleaning process. The following measures are suggested:

- protective, heavy-duty gloves must be worn when cleaning bioburden from instruments; and
- a gown or apron, mask, and protective goggles must be worn to protect against splashing contaminated fluid when washing instruments.

Disinfection using chemical disinfectants
General comments

The use of chemical disinfectants is controversial and should be limited.

Manual or mechanical cleaning is required before disinfection to reduce the load of pathogenic micro-organisms. For example, a 10% bleach-in-water solution can be applied to bench tops or equipment contaminated by potentially infectious material. However, in most cases, cleaning with detergent and hot water is all that is required.

For instruments used in invasive procedures, disinfection by immersing the object in boiling water cannot take the place of sterilisation.

A range of chemical disinfectants is usually available in any facility. Staff using chemical disinfectants should be aware that this type of disinfectant:

- is less reliable than heat;
- must not be used for instruments intended to penetrate the skin, mucous membranes, or body tissue;
- should be used only when heat sterilisation is not available; and
- must be diluted only according to manufacturers' guidelines.

Staff must wear protective rubber gloves when using chemical disinfectants.

Problems with chemical disinfection

There are several problems with chemical disinfectants. These include:

- chemical disinfection is inadequate for high-risk or medium-risk procedures;
- disinfectants vary in their effect on different organisms;
- organic matter can inactivate disinfectants;
- disinfectants can be corrosive and damage equipment;
- hard water and incompatible detergents can inactivate disinfectants;
- micro-organisms can contaminate disinfectants;
- disinfectants can be hazardous to staff health; and
- disinfectants must be used at the correct concentration and for the correct soaking time to be effective.

Alcohol

Alcohol is appropriate for disinfecting the skin and inanimate surfaces (e.g., thermometers), but does not kill spores and is not appropriate for use on instruments used in invasive procedures.

Chlorhexidine

Chlorhexidine is appropriate for disinfection of skin and mucous membranes. It is not recommended for use on inanimate surfaces or contaminated instruments.

Gluteraldehyde[6]

Gluteraldehydes should not be used in residential-care facilities because of its high toxicity and staff should be aware of the precautions associated with its use. Glutaraldehyde has been used in the health industry for many years in 1–2% solutions. It has a specific role in the 'high-level' disinfection of medical, surgical and dental equipment that is unsuitable for high temperature sterilising. In particular, glutaraldehyde solution is used to disinfect endoscopes and fibre-optic instruments that can be damaged by other disinfection procedures.

Occupational health-and-safety guidelines must be strictly followed when using this agent. Incorrect use or dilution can:

- damage instruments;
- cause adverse skin and respiratory reactions in staff members; and
- adversely affect the environment after its disposal.

Precautions must be undertaken in using gluteraldehyde. These include:

- use only in a well-ventilated room with an operating extractor fan;
- wear protective clothing (such as goggles and masks);
- use impervious gloves; and
- ensure the solution is stored in sealed labelled containers.

Hypochlorite

Because hypochlorite will not penetrate organic matter, the product is appropriate for use only on surfaces that have been cleaned. Hypochlorites can cause rust and corrosion on metal surfaces.

Hot water disinfection

Even under strictly controlled conditions, boiling instruments in water will not kill all bacterial spores, and will therefore not sterilise instruments. However, the process does provide a high degree of disinfection.

To disinfect instruments, boiling must be maintained for 20 minutes after the last instrument is added. Because boiling will not achieve sterilisation, this process can be used only for instruments not intended to penetrate the skin, mucous membranes, or other tissues.

Sterilisation[7]
General comments

An item is either sterile or not; items cannot be classed as 'almost' or 'partially' sterile.

Sterilisation and monitoring must comply with Australian/New Zealand Standard, AS/NZS 4187.[8] Sterilisation can be achieved only by monitoring the use of properly functioning sterilisers. In an aged-care facility this is likely to be by steam under pressure (e.g., in a steriliser).

Types of sterilisers
Autoclaves[9]

The most likely method of sterilisation available to residential-care staff is a benchtop steriliser. Management must ensure that instructions for operating sterilisers are displayed in a prominent position, and staff who operate sterilisers must follow the manufacturer's instructions.

The correct sterilising process is:

- a minimum of 121°C for 15 minutes; or
- a minimum of 126°C for 10 minutes.

Using material that is believed to be sterile when, in fact, it is not, places residents at significant risk of infection. The effectiveness of the sterilisation process should therefore be checked frequently and regularly, using the Australian/New Zealand Standard, AS/NZS 4187, as a guideline. A variety of testing kits are now available, which simplifies this process.

Ultraviolet sterilisers

These units might maintain the sterility of objects already sterilised, but cannot achieve sterilisation. Ultraviolet sterilisers are therefore not recommended for instruments required for use in sterile procedures.

Microwave ovens

Although a high temperature is rapidly achieved, microwave ovens have a limited effect on micro-organisms and are not recommended for instruments that are to be used in sterile procedures.

Pressure cookers

Pressure cookers produce steam under pressure. However, the temperature reached and the quality of the steam cannot be controlled. Pressure cookers are therefore not recommended for processing instruments to be used in sterile procedures.

Storage and packaging of sterile equipment

Unless sterilised items are properly cared for, there is no way of guaranteeing that sterility will be maintained. All sterile items, whether processed on site or commercially prepared, must be stored and handled in a manner that maintains the integrity of the packaging and prevents contamination. The following recommendations are made:

- Instruments can be processed and stored in sterilising bags. However, the bags must be sealed properly using heat sealers and indicator tape. The packaging will fail if other tape, pins, or staples are used.
- Ideally, the sterile items should be stored in a dry, sterile container.
- The sterile storage area should be clearly indicated.
- The sterile storage area should be dedicated to sterile items only.
- The sterile storage area must be maintained free of dust, insects, and vermin.
- All items must be stored 250 mm above floor level and 440 mm from ceiling fixtures.
- Sterile items must be protected from direct sunlight.
- Before use, check that the indicator tape has changed colour during processing.

Sterile packaged instruments and items should not be used if:

- instruments have been incorrectly wrapped;
- the package is damaged or opened;
- the package is wet, or becomes wet, after the process is complete;
- the packaged instrument comes into contact with a dirty surface (for example, the floor); or
- there is no indication that the packaged instrument has been through the sterilising process.

Equipment processed off-site[10]

After use, equipment to be processed at another facility must be properly cleaned and placed in a container with a secure lid, ready for transporting. In some cases the equipment will be bagged before transport.

Materials should be transported in a clean vehicle. After the sterilisation process, the items must be placed in a separate, clean, sealed container for return.

The processing facility should forward copies of quality activities performed as part of the sterilisation process in order to demonstrate quality improvement and compliance with appropriate standards.

When returned to the facility, the equipment must be handled and stored in a way that maintains sterility. Nursing home management must establish an agreement with the external provider clearly stating which party is responsible for the sterility of equipment processed off-site.

2. Resident care articles and equipment

The type and state of equipment used for resident care has a significant impact on residents' risk of infection. The following information will help staff to make decisions in selecting and handling resident equipment with a view to minimising the risk of cross-infection.

Procedural equipment

As noted above in the discussion on decontamination, reusable resident-care equipment must be cleaned after each use, and equipment that has been exposed to infected or potentially infected biological substances must be decontaminated (according to the manufacturer's guidelines) before reuse. In addition:

- all articles and equipment exposed to biological substances (e.g., lifting machine straps) must be washed free of organic material before decontamination;
- trolleys must be cleaned after use;
- sterile trays and sterile gloves should be used for aseptic procedures;
- disposable equipment, and articles heavily contaminated with body fluids, must be placed in designated infectious-waste containers and sent for incineration; and
- medication and diluent used in intramuscular injections, eye drops, and dressing materials must be used before their expiry dates.

Thermometers

- Mercury thermometers must be wiped with an alcohol swab after use, cleaned in soapy water, and stored dry.
- If tympanic probe thermometers are used, the probe cover must be used only once.
- If battery-operated devices are used, a 'spacer' should separate the ear from the device, and spacers should be disposed of after each use.

Oxygen masks, cannulas, and tubing

The use of humidified oxygen is rarely recommended because the moisture can lead to chest infections in susceptible residents. However, short-term, low-rate dry oxygen therapy will not dry out bronchial mucosa.

The following precautions should be followed.

- Oxygen tubing should be attached to the flowmeter by a nipple connector, rather than directly to the oxygen humidifier.
- If humidified oxygen is ordered, sterile water or sealed and pre-sterilised commercial water packs should be used. Nebulisers should be cleaned with hot, soapy water, stored dry, and returned to the same resident.
- Suction containers need not contain any solution, and must be cleaned after each use.
- Oxygen masks, cannulas and tubing are for use by a single resident only, and must be disposed of when no longer required by that resident.

Sanitation equipment

Residents' personal equipment only needs to be rinsed after use, but equipment for common use must be cleaned and decontaminated before reuse.

Bedpans and urinals should be cleaned, disinfected, and dried after use. Mechanical flushers or pan sanitisers are preferred for processing. The mechanical process involves equipment being flushed, cleaned, and then heat disinfected by hot water or steam, at 80°C for one minute. Pan sanitisers and other equipment must be maintained at peak efficiency.

Residents' personal care
Toiletries

Standards of resident care specify that residents must have their own toiletries, including shaver, soap, comb, hairbrush, deodorant, toothbrush and toothpaste.

If working in a facility where certain resident skin creams are shared, staff members should be aware that cream in tubes is less likely to become contaminated than cream in jars or containers (from which cream is scooped out with a spatula or the fingers). Such jars must never be used for more than one resident because they act as reservoirs of infection.

Wash and vomit bowls must be cleaned in hot, soapy water after use.

Mackintoshes

Because mackintoshes are used under continence-management products they are often contaminated with urine. Mackintoshes must be washed with hot soap and water rather than spraying with disinfectant and wiping the sprayed mackintosh with a cloth to remove the urine.

Shower chairs and wheelchairs

Shower chairs must be maintained in a clean condition. The following procedures are suggested.

- Shower chairs must be cleaned with hot water and detergent after each use.
- Shower chairs might require cleaning with a disinfectant if used by a resident known to have an infection or infectious disease (for example, gastroenteritis).

A common problem is that this task can become 'nobodies responsibility'—and consequently rarely carried out. Management must ensure that cleaning shower chairs and wheelchairs is designated in particular position descriptions.

Single-use products

A single-use product is a product that is designed and made to be used once only—and then discarded. A single-use product used by only one resident can be used by that resident more than once.

To minimise infection and cross infection, staff must follow the manufacturers' specifications with regard to products for single use or use by a single resident. Designated single-use products must not be reprocessed under any circumstances because reprocessing will cause deterioration or malfunction of the product, and the manufacturer will not take any responsibility for liability.

Pharmaceutical products

Lotions must be used in dilutions recommended by the manufacturer, and must be used for their stated purpose only. The use-by dates on all pharmaceutical products must be strictly observed to minimise the risk of bacterial contamination of the product.

Skin preparation[11]

Disinfectant for skin preparation should be dispensed in single-unit dose packs or decanted from the original container into a sterile container for use with individual residents. Decanted fluid remaining in the sterile container at the end of each procedure must be discarded and the container must be resterilised before reuse (or discarded if it is disposable).

The time allowed for skin disinfection should be at least two (preferably five) minutes. Skin can be disinfected with any of the following preparations:

- 70% w/w ethyl alcohol;
- 80% v/v ethyl alcohol;
- 60% v/v isopropyl alcohol;
- alcoholic (isopropyl and ethyl) formulations of 0.5–4.0% w/v chlorhexidine; or
- aqueous or alcoholic povidine-iodine (1% w/v available iodine).

Note: w/w and v/v indicate dilution; the terms stand for 'weight-for-weight' and 'volume-for-volume' respectively.

Topical preparations

Creams, lotions and drops should be used only on the resident for whom they were prescribed.

Gloves might be required for application of creams or lotions—depending on:

- the nature of the product;
- whether the condition for which the product was prescribed is infectious; and
- whether the staff member has intact skin on his or her hands.

Staff members must wash their hands before and after the procedure (whether they have worn gloves or not).

Eye drops

The following procedures are recommended when using eye drops.

- Eye toilets should be done before instillation of drops.
- Staff members must wash their hands before carrying out the procedure. It is not neccessary to wear gloves.
- Staff must ensure there is no contact between the dropper and the conjunctiva.
- Eye drops must be used before their use-by date.

Solutions commonly used for procedures

Aqueous chlorhexidine: This is used as a cleaning agent before insertion of a urinary catheter.

Bleach: The use of bleach is discouraged from an occupational health-and-safety point of view. In addition, its effectiveness has not been established.

Chlorhexidine/alcohol hand rub: This can be used as a hand-cleanser between hand-washings.

Chlorhexidine hand wash: This is used in a 2% solution for clinical hand-washing.

Hydrogen peroxide: This can be used, diluted, in certain types of mouth care. It is rarely used for wound debridement.

Methylated spirits: This is not effective as a disinfectant.

Normal saline: This is a useful solution for wound irrigation and mouth care.

Povidine-iodine: Current research suggests that povidine iodine should be used only as a preoperative skin preparation and on superficial skin lesions. It should not be used for packing wounds because it can actually inhibit wound healing.[12]

Sodium hypochlorite 500 ppm (parts per million): In 1994, 'Milton' (a commercial sodium hypochlorite solution) was recategorised by the Therapeutic Goods Administration as 'not approved' for use in surgery or any type of wound irrigation or disinfection of tissue. However, it is still approved for disinfecting inanimate objects (such as equipment or work surfaces), and can be used for soaking equipment when no other form of disinfection or sterilisation is available. It should be used for blood and body substance spills if there is a risk of contamination.

Drug therapy

Local anaesthetic and other injectable substances

Because injection needles penetrate the skin, extreme care must be taken to prevent contamination and cross-infection from staff to residents, and from residents to staff.

Injections must always be given with sterile needles and syringes, and the utmost care must be taken when disposing of the used needle.

When injectable local anaesthetic is required, the most effective way to avoid cross-infection is by using single-dose vials. A sterile needle and sterile syringe must be used for withdrawing fluid, and both the needle and syringe must be discarded after one use.[13] This is particularly necessary if the required agent is only available in a multidose vial.

Oral medication

Oral medication must be dispensed hygienically. Tablets should be tipped into the lid of the container, rather than into the dispenser's hand.

Spoons for liquids should be used for only one resident and then washed. Staff members should wash their hands before attending to the next resident.

Using syringes to dispense suspensions should be discouraged unless the syringe is used for a single resident and the syringe is cleaned appropriately between doses.

Antibiotic therapy

Full courses of prescribed antibiotics must be completed to ensure that the infecting organism does not become resistant to the drug, and that the infection resolves completely. Consideration should be given to using the Antibiotic Guidelines.[14]

3. Environmental services: cleaning the kitchen and laundry

Cleaning services

General

Cleaning ensures that the care environment is as free as possible from micro-organisms—thereby reducing a source of infection for residents and staff. Because the physical environment is contaminated with micro-organisms, the work of the environmental services worker is vital to preventing cross infection. Pathogenic micro-organisms can remain viable in the environment for long periods after their release from host tissues (for example, VRE in dust[15]). Regular and thorough environmental cleaning is necessary to reduce the number of microorganisms present and to prevent reservoirs of micro-organisms from being established.

Care must also be taken to minimise the dispersal of organisms while cleaning. The method of cleaning must therefore be chosen carefully to prevent redistributing soil or micro-organisms. Because some dispersal of dust and organisms is inevitable during cleaning, cleaners should not work in an area where a procedure (such as a wound dressing) is being performed.

All stores and equipment must be stored off the floor to allow easy access and appropriate cleaning.

Organising cleaning duties

Cleaning commences in the cleaners' room where equipment used for cleaning purposes should be adequately washed after use and stored dry until they are needed again.

The workflow should move methodically from high dusting to floor cleaning. The frequency of cleaning can vary from daily to a 'needs basis'—as determined by regular auditing. A documented cleaning schedule should be developed and should be available for all staff to consult. An example is shown in Table 5.2 (page 79).

As Table 5.2 suggests, the facility's cleaning schedule identifies:
- what is cleaned;
- the staff member responsible for cleaning;
- how the cleaning is to be performed;
- the frequency of cleaning; and
- the specific products and equipment to be used.

Cleaning methods

Damp-dusting

Vertical surfaces are damp-dusted when they are visibly dusty. Horizontal surfaces are dusted on a needs basis. Cleaners contribute to the fight against cross-infection if they observe the following infection-control suggestions.

- Use a 'rinse-and-wring' method with a bowl of hot water and detergent.
- Remember that moisture can provide conditions for micro-organisms to thrive and grow. Therefore, drying surfaces is an essential part of the cleaning process.
- Make sure all surfaces are damp-dusted. Dust from the top to the bottom. Use smooth strokes to avoid stirring up the dust. Flicking the duster spreads micro-organisms.
- Clean the duster frequently to ensure dust is not simply moved from place to place.

Vacuuming

Floors are cleaned by a combination of vacuuming and mopping—on an established needs basis. Areas of high usage will need more frequent attention than will rarely used surfaces. Brooms should be discouraged because sweeping merely aerosolises (blows into the air in fine particles) soil and dust that contain micro-organisms, which are then deposited in another area, rather than removed.

The following procedures are recommended.

- Make sure the vacuum exhaust is filtered, so dust and dirt particles are not blown into the air. Ensure that the filter is cleared at regular intervals.
- Pick up large or sharp items safely before vacuuming, to avoid blocking or damaging the equipment.
- Spot clean any spills before vacuuming.

Table 5.2 Sample cleaning schedule

Item or area	Method of cleaning	Products to be used	Frequency of cleaning	Staff member
Floors (hard surface)	Vacuuming, followed by mopping	Hot water and detergent	Daily or second daily and on a needs basis	Cleaner
Floors (carpet)	Vacuuming and shampooing	Commercial carpet shampoo	Vacuum daily or second daily and shampoo on a needs basis	Cleaner
Air conditioning ducts	Vacuuming and damp dusting	Vacuum (clean filter regularly)	On a needs basis	Engineer or maintenance staff
Walls and ceilings	Washing	Hot water and detergent (disinfect only if contamination with body substance has occurred)	On a needs basis when a build-up of visible soilage become obvious	Cleaner
Doors	Washing	Detergent and water	Daily cleaning of handles, spot clean door as needs	Cleaner
High dusting, including removal of cobwebs	Dusting with extension duster, or vacuuming	Dry dust	At least monthly, and on a needs basis	Cleaner

Table 5.2 (cont.)

Item or area	Method of cleaning	Products to be used	Frequency of cleaning	Staff member
Showers recesses	Rubbing with a cloth* and cleaning solution	Hot water and detergent. Bleach may be used as a whitener Cream cleanser can be used for stains and marks	Every day, but more frequently if necessary	Cleaner
Washbasins and toilet bowls	Rubbing with a cloth,* scrubbing with a toilet brush**	Hot water and detergent. Bleach may be used as a whitener. Cream cleaner can be used for stains and marks	At least daily, more often if contaminated with body fluids	Cleaner
Baths	Rubbing with a cloth* and cleaning solution	Hot water and detergent. Bleach may be used as a whitener. Cream cleanser can be used for stains and marks and to remove scum	After each resident use	Cleaner and nurse (according to position description)
Spa Baths	Rubbing with a cloth* and cleaning solution	Must be disinfected after each use with a commercial chlorine-releasing agent, to a level of 5–10ppm (parts per million)	After each resident use	Cleaner and nurse (according to position description)

Table 5.2 (cont.)

Item or area	Method of cleaning	Products to be used	Frequency of cleaning	Staff member
Pillows	Wipe down plastic covers	Hot water wash with detergent. Clean entire pillow according to manufacturer's instructions	On a needs basis	Nurse and laundryhand
Macintosh on bed	Wipe down or may be laundered	Hot water and detergent. May be dried on the washing line	Daily and when necessary after contamination with body fluids	Nurse
Mattress Bed frames, walking frames and bed rails	Wipe down plastic cover Wipe down with a cloth* and cleaning solution	Hot water and detergent Hot water and detergent	On a needs basis. Before use with a new resident and when contaminated with body fluids	Cleaner and nurse (according to position description)
Lifting machine and weighing chair	Wipe down with a cloth* and cleaning solution	Hot water and detergent	On a needs basis. Webbing straps should be laundered on a scheduled basis and when necessary after contamination with body fluids	Cleaner and nurse (according to position description)

Table 5.2 (cont.)

Item or area	Method of cleaning	Products to be used	Frequency of cleaning	Staff member
Pillows	Wipe down plastic covers	Hot water wash with detergent. Clean entire pillow according to manufacturer's instructions	On a needs basis	Nurse and laundryhand
Macintosh on bed	Wipe down or may be laundered	Hot water and detergent. May be dried on the washing line	Daily and when necessary after contamination with body fluids	Nurse
Mattress Bed frames, walking frames and bed rails	Wipe down plastic cover Wipe down with a cloth* and cleaning solution	Hot water and detergent Hot water and detergent	On a needs basis. Before use with a new resident and when contaminated with body fluids	Cleaner and nurse (according to position description)
Lifting machine and weighing chair	Wipe down with a cloth* and cleaning solution	Hot water and detergent	On a needs basis. Webbing straps should be laundered on a scheduled basis and when necessary after contamination with body fluids	Cleaner and nurse (according to position description)

Table 5.2 (cont.)

Food preparation surfaces	Washing	Hot water and detergent. May be disinfected with sodium hypochlorite 500 ppm	At least once per shift	Food services staff
Storage rooms	Wipe down all surfaces	Hot water and detergent	Three monthly and on a needs basis	Cleaner
Outside barbecue and waste storage areas (including bins)	weeping and scrubbing surfaces with brush	Hot water and detergent	At least monthly, and on a needs basis	Maintenance staff

* washcloths must be washed or discarded at the end of each shift and on a needs basis
** toilet brushes should be flushed with water after use, and stored dry

Damp-mopping

The most effective way to damp-mop is to use hot water and detergent. Ensure that the water is changed frequently—because cold water will disperse dirt, dust and micro-organisms (rather than collect them).

The following procedures are recommended.

- Rinse and wring the mop frequently.
- Change the water frequently (for example, every six rooms and at the end of the shift. Dirty water should be disposed of into the designated sink in the cleaners' room or dirty utility room.
- Fixed mop heads are very difficult to clean. Detachable mop heads are more appropriate for use because they can be laundered daily on a hot-wash cycle and dried in the clothes drier or in the sun before reuse.
- Mops must not be left soaking in buckets of water when not in use.
- Buckets should be cleaned frequently, and stored dry when not in use.

Cleaning solutions
Storage

It is common for large quantities of cleaning solutions to be stored in residential facilities. All cleaning solutions (including laundry solutions) are potentially harmful chemicals. It is important that such chemicals are stored and handled according to the safety data sheets supplied by chemical companies.

To comply with occupational health and safety requirements:

- safety data sheets must be up to date and available in the work area;
- all chemicals must be clearly and correctly labelled; and
- an eye wash should be readily available for use in the case of chemical splash.

Choice of solution

There are many cleaning solutions on the market and the choice can be bewildering. Many of the solutions are unnecessarily strong and expensive. The discussion below will assist managers to make an appropriate selection.

But first, a word about the use of spray bottles in cleaning routines. Spray bottles are often used for cleaning. This practice is a poor method of cleaning because a damp or dry cloth is then used to simply 'join the dots', or spread the spray that has landed on the surface to be cleaned.

In addition:

- cold sprays do not necessarily kill germs;
- the dilution is rarely correct because spray bottles are often 'topped up' with water;
- disinfectants are easily deactivated in clear bottles and have a short shelf life;
- spray bottle nozzles are rarely cleaned and can therefore harbour micro-organisms;
- much of the chemical is aerosolised and sprayed into the atmosphere (instead of making contact with the surface to be cleaned); and
- spray bottles can create an occupational health-and-safety risk.

A more effective method is to use a container of detergent and hot water, immerse a cloth, wring it out, and then wash the area using old-fashioned 'elbow grease'.

Detergents

A detergent is a chemical wetting agent that acts as a degreaser and makes cleaning easier. The mechanical action of the cleaning, combined with the product, provides effective cleaning. A detergent does not kill micro-organisms. However, in combination with hot water, it can be very effective for reducing the number of micro-organisms on the surface or item to be cleaned. Detergents are not expensive and are widely available.

When using detergent in a cleaning routine, be aware of the following two points:

- the detergent and water mixture must be changed frequently to maintain the water temperature and avoid cross infection;
- detergent and disinfectant should never be mixed together (unless recommended by the supplier) because the effect of one often cancels out the other.

Disinfectants

As previously noted, disinfectants are not cleaners. Rather, they are chemical agents that are capable of killing some micro-organisms. Disinfectants must be used in the recommended concentration.

If the solution is too weak it:

- will not kill micro-organisms; and
- can cause the user to work unnecessarily hard to gain the desired result; and
- can lead to accumulation of soiling on surfaces and repetition of work.

If the solution is too strong it can result in:

- unwanted deposits and smears;
- unpleasant and possibly toxic fumes; and
- corrosion or damage to surface coatings.

Unfortunately disinfectants are often over-used or used inappropriately. No disinfectant is 100% effective. The outcome will therefore rely on:

- effective cleaning being carried out first to remove surplus dirt and dust.
- correct dilution of the disinfectant; and
- allowing 3–10 minutes' contact time, as specified by the manufacturer.

Cleaning flower vase water and potplants

The water in vases and soil from pot plants can harbour harmful micro-organisms. Changing flower water and tending to pot plants must be done daily to reduce the likelihood of cross infection. Whoever is assigned this duty must wash hands carefully afterwards to avoid spreading infection.

Cleaning to control Legionnaires' Disease[16]

The spread of Legionnaires' disease due to the presence of *Legionella pneumophilia* is unlikely if air-cooling and hot-water systems are regularly and adequately maintained.

Care of air-conditioning cooling towers and hot water systems

Because of the infection-control danger posed by poorly maintained water systems, maintenance of cooling towers and hot-water systems is governed by strict regulations (e.g., in Victoria, Section 25 of the *Health [Infectious Diseases] Regulations* 1990). In addition, phone advice can be obtained from the local health department.

New cooling towers require cleaning and disinfection before commissioning, with water samples taken 24–48 hours later to check for bacteria. Most existing cooling towers have been designed for easy cleaning and maintenance. Fitting chemical pumps that continuously circulate biocides can enhance the cleanliness of the water. Biocides are chemical agents designed to kill micro-organisms.

Adequate maintenance of cooling towers includes the following monthly cleaning and inspection routines by specialist external contractors:

- clean and flush out the holding basin;
- check biocide levels from the automatic dosing pumps;
- clean the filter pad and strainers, replacing if there is any sign of deterioration

- check and adjust the water pump float valve;
- check the fan belts and bearings;
- check all flexible joints for leaks;
- check the overflow drain;
- check the operation of the dump valve;
- samples of water from the towers and hot-water systems are tested for Legionella;

In addition to the above monthly checks, an annual check should be carried out, before summer, during which cooling towers are washed and cleaned.

Guidelines also recommend a regimen for checking and maintaining hot water systems and showers.[17]

Food services[18, 19]

Could this happen in your facility's kitchen?

1. The food services assistant, wearing gloves and serving food, takes off her cap, rearranges her hair, puts on her cap again and goes back to serving food—without changing gloves or washing hands.

2. There is meat thawing on the same tray as Pavlova.

3. The chef arrives on duty, rearranges cooked breakfast foods, uses the phone, flicks through the phone book—and then goes back to the food without washing his hands.

Staff practices

Food contaminated with micro-organisms is capable of causing disease among residents and staff. Hygienic procedures designed to avoid infecting food are essential during the preparation and storage of food. The most important food-handling procedure is hand-washing.

Staff with the following infections should not handle food:

- acute gastroenteritis (caused by *Salmonella* or other organisms);
- cholera or dysentery;
- hepatitis A and E;
- tapeworm;
- active tuberculosis;
- the common cold; or
- influenza.

Staff members returning from leave after being diagnosed with any of these conditions should provide a medical certificate stating that they are free from infection and fit to return to work.

Infection control in the kitchen
Best practice
- The kitchen-cleaning schedule is strictly adhered to.
- Stock is rotated to ensure 'first-in' is first used.
- Contamination of cooked food by raw food is avoided by using separate, designated chopping boards for cooked and raw foods.
- Prepared food is always covered.
- Breakfast foods (e.g., cereal) are covered when plated.
- Meals are served and delivered to residents in as short a time as possible.
- Fly-wire screens are present and intact on all kitchen windows.
- Staff members, other than kitchen staff, are discouraged from entering the kitchen.
- A separate sink is provided for hand washing.

Safe food storage
- Store all foods off the floor.
- Store dry foods in clean, dry and sealed containers in areas that are well ventilated and vermin-proof.
- Store flour and cereals in metal or plastic, sealed containers to protect the food from mice, rats and damp. Use a separate scoop for each container.
- Check canned goods for rust, splits, dents, leaks and 'use-by' dates.
- Treat opened cans as fresh food.
- Store vegetables on racks to allow adequate air circulation.
- Check any vegetables held for more than a few days for deterioration.
- Store fresh fruit separately because apples and citrus fruits can taint other foods. Avoid crushing fruit because this makes the fruit prone to deterioration and mould growth.
- Store milk in the refrigerator.
- Separate raw and cooked foods:
- If only one refrigerator is available, cooked foods should be stored above raw foods, so there is no leakage on to, and possible contamination of, cooked food by raw food.

- Uncooked meats should be sealed in plastic wrapping to avoid leakage.
- Food should be returned to the refrigerator within two hours of cooking and kept no longer than three days.
- Stored, cooked food should be dated.

Refrigeration

The availability of modern refrigerator storage has done much to increase the availability of fresh foods. However, refrigeration of foods must be carefully monitored to ensure that the food is maintained at temperatures that discourage the multiplication of any micro-organisms already present in the food.

- Refrigerator temperature should be maintained between 3° and 4°C.
- Avoid overloading the refrigerator (because this will decrease the circulation of cold air).
- Never refreeze food that has been thawed.
- Milk and milk products must be kept refrigerated.

Cook-chill

Cook-chill is a method of preparing, plating, and refrigerating large quantities of food in advance of meal times. The chilled, plated food can be transported to the site of consumption and reheated or 'regenerated' in a special trolley over a prescribed period of time.

Cook-chill is used in many facilities. However, because of the extended process of preparation and storage before consumption, food services staff should:

- store and reheat the food strictly in accordance with the process recommendations;
- ensure that equipment is serviced and checked regularly; and
- promptly report any equipment malfunctions (for example timers).

Care of crockery and cutlery

- meal trays and dirty dishes should be removed from resident-care areas as soon as possible.
- Crockery and cutlery must be scraped and food scraps placed in plastic disposal bags before the dishes are washed.
- To ensure a temperature of 80°C or above, the temperature of dishwashers must be checked frquently as part of surveillance and routine maintenance.
- Detergent must be used with every dishwasher load.

- If dishes are washed manually, use hot soapy water, change it frequently, and follow with a hot water rinse.
- Meal trays must be washed with detergent.
- Eating utensils are adequately cleaned if they have been washed effectively in detergent and hot water.

Cleaning the kitchen

- Keep work areas clean.
- Scrub wood, marble and other food contact surfaces at least daily with hot soapy water.
- Clean shelves and storage areas weekly, or more often if necessary, to ensure no food particles collect there.
- Keep pantries scrupulously clean and free from vermin.
- Cover grease traps or drains.

Food safety plans

It appears likely, as has happened in Victoria[20] and some other states, that all facilities will be required to develop a food-safety plan that includes hazard analysis and control points.

Such a plan includes documentation that:

- identifies potential and actual hazards and problems;
- identifies control measures for each potential hazard;
- specifies how to address specific problems;
- provides methods of supervision and monitoring of controls, including auditing; and
- specifies the food hygiene training provided for food-services staff.

Laundry services[21]

Soiled linen is a bacterial reservoir of micro-organisms and a potential source of infection. Laundering linen does not guarantee decontamination—unless the laundering is effective and meets infection control standards. If laundry standards are not met and maintained, micro-organisms can survive the laundering process and cause nosocomial infection.

Laundering residents' personal items of clothing

Ensure that routine washing, drying, and ironing procedures are adequate for personal items of laundry that are not contaminated by body fluids.

Wash temperature

- All linen should be regarded as potentially infectious. A cold wash is therefore not acceptable for communal clothes washing.
- The correct temperature range and time for a hot-water wash is 70–85°C for 12 minutes.
- A small laundry dryer temperature cannot be relied on to kill micro-organisms. (Note that in large commercial laundries, the dryer temperature is approximately 180°C.)

Laundry solutions

- The correct amount of laundry detergent must be used (correct dosing). Chemical companies are obliged to provide regular product reports about correct dosing, pH levels, and other information relevant to the occupational health and safety of laundry workers. Incorrect dosing can result in ineffective washing or a build-up of residual chemical on the linen.
- Solutions should be used in the machines at appropriate temperature ranges. Cold water detergents should be used with hot water at 70–85°C, but staff mebers will require advice on the correct procedure from the chemical supplier. Bleach is not activated until 60°C.
- Chlorine bleach is stable when stored, but is volatile when handled. This can damage clothing fabrics. Contact the supplier for handling, storing, and dosage levels.

Laundry equipment

- Laundry machinery must be routinely maintained to ensure efficient operation. This includes regular changing of filters and checking of hoses for corrosion and leakage. The back of the machines must be wiped free of lint and dusted regularly.
- Laundry trolleys used for storing soiled linen must be cleaned thoroughly before being used to transport clean linen.
- The laundry floor must be cleaned daily. If a laundry contractor is used, the facility's management must ensure that the contractor's practices comply with infection control guidelines, specifically, AS/NZS 4146: 2000.[22]

Sluicing

The practice of using tap water under pressure to remove or hose off faecal matter from soiled linen is not acceptable. The practice poses occupational health-and-safety risks for staff (due to splattering of biological material).

The following suggestions are effective alternatives to sluicing:

- If excess excreta are disposed into the sluice, a well-maintained washing machine will wash the linen adequately without adversely affecting the machine, or other linen in the wash.
- All soiled items can be washed in one load after carefully removing excess excreta from the linen with a spatula or gloved hand.
- Sluicing machines are available. These machines have wider drainage holes to drain solid particles after a 'sluicing cycle' in the normal wash.
- If sluicing is practised, full protective apparel must be worn.

Handling used linen

- As part of standard precautions, all staff members handling heavily soiled linen should wear gloves.
- Linen must never be placed on the floor because of the risk of depositing body fluids on the floor.
- Staff should take care not to gather up equipment or residents' personal possessions with soiled linen. Non-linen items (e.g., a resident's watch) accidentally placed in the linen container will require decontamination.
- Used linen must be deposited in linen skips, preferably at the resident's bedside.
- Linen must be transported in designated linen bags (e.g., Kylies or Buddies in Kylie or Buddy bags). Additional segregation of used linen into specific bags might be required, depending on the laundry practices in the facility.
- Linen skips must be changed when they are two-thirds full (to avoid potential contamination from overflow, and to facilitate manoeuvrability).
- In case there is a sharp inside, linen bags must not be pushed down by human hands, and must be braced against the body. They must be dragged across the floor in case the bag splits.
- When full bags are tied and placed for collection, care must be taken not to contaminate the outside of the bag.
- The use of standard precautions has superseded the need for double bagging of so-called 'infectious linen'.
- Linen chutes are discouraged because they are difficult to clean and because linen bags can tear on the way down. Any fine spray of biological fluids when the bag lands on the lower floor will contaminate the immediate environment. Chutes can also be wrongly used for rubbish or other hazardous material.
- Hands must be washed after contact with used linen.
- Linen waiting to be collected by an external service provider must be stored in a secure weatherproof environment.

Protective clothing for laundry staff

Laundry staff members must take care when handling clothes and garments that are contaminated by blood or body fluids. They should wear gloves to handle linen in the laundry, use additional protective clothing (such as plastic aprons and protective eye wear) when indicated, and place linen directly into the washing machine.

Managing clean linen

- Clean linen must be stored in a clean, dry area and kept separate from used linen.
- Hands must be washed before contact with clean linen.
- Clean linen should be handled as little as possible.
- Stored clean linen must be rotated regularly to ensure linen is not stored for excessive periods of time (creating a build-up of dust), and that stock wears evenly.

3. Pest control and waste management

Pest Control

General

Pests spread infection. The most common pests in residential facilities are rats, mice, ants, cockroaches, and flies.

The individual contribution of staff members to the elimination of pest infestation is vital. Unless staff members report sightings of pests, no action can be taken. Management must encourage staff members to report sighting of pests (by, for example, supplying a centrally located book for this purpose.

Scheduled routine surveillance of the facility by a pest-control service is recommended. The service provider must have access to reports of pest sightings and supply a report after each visit, including:

- what was discovered;
- how it was treated; and
- details of proposed follow up.

Signs and sites of infestation

Watch out for:

- damaged, stored goods;
- gnaw marks on pipes, timber, and plastic;
- smear marks on rafters and walls; and
- rodent droppings.

Typical locations for pests

Typical locations for pests include:

- in cracks and crevices (for example, behind broken wall tiles, sinks, and skirting boards);
- beneath refrigerators or ovens;
- in boiler rooms;
- in and around service ducts;
- in food-storage areas; and
- in kitchen grease traps and waste-disposal areas.

Waste management[23]

General

Approved containers must be available for the disposal of:

- used sharps;
- biological waste and contaminated material (e.g., used dressings); and
- discarded, single-use equipment.

In Australia, waste-disposal bags have been standardised in colour to allow ready identification.[24] Using the correct colour-coding assists in safe handling and correct disposal of waste. Various colours have been assigned to different types of waste. However, for infection control in residential facilities, the following colour protocol should be sufficient:

- black for general waste; and
- yellow for clinical and potentially infectious waste.

Clinical waste

Clinical waste includes:

- clinical specimens other than urine or faeces;
- specimens of urine or faeces collected for laboratory-testing;
- swabs taken for laboratory culture;
- human tissue;
- human blood and body fluids (other than urine and faeces);
- materials or equipment containing human blood or body fluids (other than urine or faeces);
- waste from residents known to have, or suspected of having a communicable disease (AS/NZS 3816: 1998).[25]

It could be argued that the disposal of continence aids contaminated with organisms such as MRSA and VRE should be controlled by supervised landfill procedures.

Note: Urine or faecal material can be safely disposed of into the sewer.

Care of waste

The environment protection authority (EPA) in each state must license waste-disposal contractors. The facility management's responsibility for waste generated onsite continues until, and including, the actual disposal. Enquiries should therefore be made about the practices of the contractor.

In addition to monitoring the practices of contractors, management and staff must include the following waste-disposal points in their infection-control strategy.

1. Bins must be:
   - weather-safe and secure against animals or vermin;
   - emptied on a needs basis, but at least weekly; and
   - secured from public access.

2. Waste bags must:
   - never be braced against the body or dragged across the floor;
   - not be compacted by hands or feet;
   - be inspected regularly to ensure the contents are appropriate to the type of bag (especially infectious waste bags).

3. Incontinence pads, colostomy bags, and urinary drainage bags can be disposed of into the general waste for land fill (after the contents have been carefully drained into the sewer).

4. Food waste can be discarded into the general waste or through garbage-disposal units or composted.

If in doubt about any aspect of waste disposal, facility management should consult:
   - their contracted waste-disposal contractor;
   - state health department;
   - local council; or
   - the environment protection authority (EPA).

Chapter 6

Quality Management

Achieving quality in care

Infection-control policies should be coffee-stained and dog-eared—not shelved and clean. Quality management[1] focuses on achieving the highest-possible level of care and service, given the available resources. Achieving quality management in residential aged care means that all staff members adopt, and practise, a philosophy that is centred on continuous improvement of all aspects of the facility's operation.

In residential aged care, quality-management systems are a necessary prerequisite for meeting standards and gaining accreditation. All aged-care standards include three expected quality-related outcomes:[2]

- continuous improvement;
- regulatory compliance; and
- education and staff development.

Adopting a quality system involves the establishment, implementation, documentation and maintenance of quality practices in every area of the facility. This can be diagrammatically represented by a quality cycle (see Figure 6.1),[3] which demonstrates the continuous process of monitoring, assessment, action, follow-up and continuous feedback.

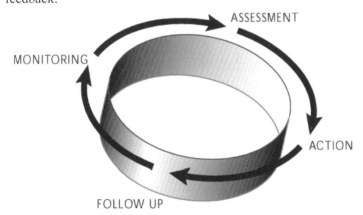

Figure 6.1 The Quality Cycle

Adapted with permission from Australian Health-Care Associates and Commonwealth Department of Health and Family Services (1997)[4]

Achieving quality requires:

- a commitment from all levels of staff, including management;
- the involvement of residents and their representatives in the quality process; and
- regular internal review of staff compliance with the facility's recommended practices.

The care and service given by staff should be equivalent to the level of care that staff members would like to receive themselves. Even when quality standards are achieved, staff and management should strive to improve further.

Quality management in infection control

Infection control is an integral component of quality improvement in health-care facilities. Quality in infection control is based on staff education, surveillance of quality practices, and a constant desire by staff and management to improve infection-control practices.

Surveillance[5]

Infection-control quality management is demonstrated by systematic and comprehensive surveillance, including documentation of: (i) nosocomial infection among residents; and (ii) staff exposure to potentially infectious material. Surveillance might be intermittent or continuous. In some cases it is planned, whereas in others it is developed in response to a specific issue of concern.

The objectives of surveillance are therefore:

- to establish a baseline, or prevalence study, of nosocomial infection in the facility; and
- to identify procedures which expose staff to infection.

Suggested surveillance activities include keeping records of:

- the number of residents with skin breaks or wounds that become infected;
- the number of residents with conjunctivitis;
- the number of residents with diarrhoea;
- the number of residents with confirmed urinary tract infections;
- antibiotic usage among residents;
- prescribers' compliance with recommended antibiotic guidelines;[6]

- observed staff compliance with standard precautions policy;
- the number of confirmed incidents of staff exposure to body fluids, and whether exposed staff complied with facility policy regarding follow up;
- waste-disposal practices (i.e., segregation, storage and transport);
- compliance with environmental cleaning practices;
- analysis of how hazardous practices in the food services area was managed; and
- analysis of how outbreaks were managed.

Benchmarking

Benchmarking is a commonly used term. However, to compare facilities' infection rates and surveillance results correctly the facilities must be similar in terms of:

- bed numbers;
- numbers of males and females living in the facilities;
- resident dependency levels; and
- degree of debilitation and rehabilitation assistance required by residents.

Infection rates can vary due to climatic changes, increased resident dependency, level of care required, and staffing levels.

Outbreak management and follow up[7]

Notification

An outbreak of an infection or infectious disease is defined as two or more cases of an identical illness occurring in a facility in a relatively short space of time.

Quality-management practices during an outbreak of infectious illness are designed to achieve swift control by assessing the risk and adopting measures to limit the outbreak. Urgent action is required to prevent further spread. During an outbreak, communication with the relevant authorities is essential. In Victoria, for example, outbreaks of infectious diseases must be reported to:

- the Public Health Unit, Department of Human Services;
- the Infectious Diseases Unit, Department of Human Services (if a notifiable disease causes the outbreak);
- the Food Safety Unit, Department of Human Services (if the outbreak is caused by a foodborne illness);
- the Water Technology Unit Department of Health and Community Services (if the outbreak is caused by a waterborne illness);
- the regional environmental health officer;
- the local government environmental health officer; and
- the residents' medical practitioners.

Although such a list might seem daunting, it is usually more efficient to report outbreaks to the relevant authorities as soon as possible and gain assistance—rather than trying to manage them inhouse without adequate resources and backup.

See Appendix A for a list of Australian and New Zealand health departments.

See Appendix B for a list of Australian and New Zealand notifiable diseases.

Immediate response to an outbreak

Carefully compiled documentation of the outbreak is invaluable in assisting authorities deal efficiently with the outbreak.

Gastrointestinal outbreak

A foodborne outbreak is caused by bacteria or viruses that are acquired by: (i) ingestion of contaminated food or water; or (ii) exposure to infected faeces or vomit. The signs and symptoms vary with each individual case, but can include some or all of the following:

- diarrhoea;
- abdominal cramps;
- nausea;
- vomiting;
- headache; and
- fever.

Immediate action consists of:

1. Cease ingestion of the suspected source (i.e., infected food or water).

2. Isolate and retain samples of the suspected source for possible examination.

3. Separate residents with signs and symptoms from those with no signs and symptoms.

4. Establish whether any staff members have been unwell.

5. Send any sick staff members home.

6. Prepare a list of all residents and staff with symptoms of illness, including days and times of onset.

7. Be alert for new cases.

8. Be wary of accepting any new residents.

9. Suspend routine environmental cleaning until approved by investigators.

Follow up action consist of:

1. Ensure all contaminated food or fluids are disposed of carefully and correctly.

2. Ensure equipment, benches, floors, and toilets are thoroughly cleaned.

3. Instruct sick staff members not to return until they are symptom-free for 48 hours.

4. Liaise with investigating authorities and commence recommended strategies (such as water treatment).

Non-gastrointestinal outbreaks

In non-gastrointestinal outbreaks, such as measles and whooping cough, individual cases will present with various signs and symptoms. If an infection is suspected, the following steps should be observed.

Immediate action consists of:

1. Contact the local public health unit for advice.

2. Separate residents with signs and symptoms from those with no symptoms.

3. Establish whether any staff members have been unwell.

4. Send any sick staff members home.

5. Prepare a list of all residents and staff with symptoms of illness (including days and times of onset).

6. Be alert for new cases.

7. Be wary of accepting any new residents.

Follow up action consist of:

1. Ensure appropriate infection control practices are in place.

2. Avoid risk of cross infection.

3. Vaccinate residents who have not been vaccinated (if applicable).

4. Monitor the situation to identify any further cases.

Documented quality management

At this point it is worth recalling that infection-control strategies in residential facilities are directed towards maintaining and improving resident care, protecting staff, and providing a safe environment. An essential quality-management, infection-control strategy for any residential facility includes developing a system that contains the following components:

- a program to monitor staff infection-control practices;
- a systematic method of collecting data regarding infection rates;
- a method of meaningfully analysing the collected data;
- a process for disseminating results-based information to staff;
- a method of involving staff in planning any necessary change to work practices.

Practical approaches to infection control

The following set of tables provides some examples of documented infection-control quality-management monitoring systems.

The first table (Table 6.1) defines an infection-control quality-plan that identifies areas and practices that need to be assessed and reviewed to establish compliance with recommended practices and parameters for improvement. The plan cites the activity, its aims, strategies for implementation, and the methods used to collect information, areas of responsibility and liaison, defined time targets and proposed outcome evaluation and the use to be made of the information.

The following nine tables are audit tools relating to staff practices. They are:

Table 6.2 Handwashing practices audit;

Table 6.3 Linen care audit;

Table 6.4 Disposal of sharps audit;

Table 6.5 Single-use items audit;

Table 6.6 Staff questionnaires;

Table 6.7 Podiatry survey audit;

Table 6.8 Hairdressing and beauty therapy audit;

Table 6.9 Cleaning audit;

Table 6.10 Storage of sterile stock audit;

Table 6.11 An example of a completed quality-assurance activity report of linen care using the linen-care audit table.

The final four tables are monitoring sheets that document or identify established infections within the facility. They are:

Table 6.12 Infection-control worksheet;

Table 6.13 Infection-control monthly statistics;

Table 6.14 Infection-control action sheet;

Table 6.15 Infection-control yearly statistics.

Table 6.1 Lornadoone infection-control quality plan 2003

Activity	Aim of activity	Strategies for implementation & methods used to gain information	Responsibility & liaisons	Target month	Proposed Outcome evaluation & intended use of information
Monthly Infection Surveillance	To monitor infections within the facility	– Pathology reports – Nursing staff reporting – Resident histories	IC Rep & Management	Monthly	– Implement change if indicated
Evaluation of Catering Services re Food Safety Plan	To review staff and facility compliance with Food Act 1984 amended 1998	– Food Act / Food safety plan – Review of department – Observation staff practice	IC Rep, Management & staff	Monthly	– Staff compliance with recommended guidelines – Risk control
Monitoring medication refrigerators	To establish temperature maintenance as per recommendations	– Surveillance results – Maintenance records	IC Rep & Management	Monthly	– Compliance with recommended guidelines – Risk control
Blood Exposure Injuries	To monitor staff injuries To identify risks	– Staff incident reports – Pathology results	IC Rep & Management	Monthly	– Monitor incidence – Implement strategies as indicated to minimise risk.

Table 6.1 Lornadoone infection-control quality plan 2003 (cont.)

Activity	Aim of activity	Strategies for implementation & methods used to gain information	Responsibility & liaisons	Target month	Proposed outcome evaluation & intended use of information
QA Plan	To plan activities for the year as part of ongoing review of the infection control program	– Previous plans – Surveillance reports – Results of previous audits	IC Rep & Management	January	– Monitor quality improvement activities – Implement change as required
Manual Review	To review Infection control manual	– Consultation with staff – Standards and guidelines	IC Rep, Management & staff	January / February	– Compliance with recommended guidelines
Sharps Audit	To assess compliance with documented guidelines	– Documented guidelines – EPA guidelines – AS/NZS 3816:1998	IC Rep & Management	January July	– Compliance with recommended guidelines – Risk minimisation
Summaries of nosocomial infections and Blood Exposure Injuries	To review on an annual basis infection rates and blood exposure incidents	– Monthly infection surveillance reports – Staff incident reports – Pathology results	IC Rep & Management	February	– Compare yearly rates – Implement change as indicated – Implement risk control

Table 6.1 Lornadoone infection-control quality plan 2003 (cont.)

	Objective	Standard	Responsibility	Timeframe	Outcome
Single Use	To review compliance with Single Use policy	– AS 4187–1998 – Documented guidelines – Observation	IC Rep & Management	February August	– Compliance with recommended guidelines – Risk control
Waste audit	To assess compliance with documented guidelines	– Documented guidelines – EPA guidelines – AS/NZS 3816:1998	IC Rep, Management & staff	February August	– Compliance with recommended guidelines – Risk minimisation
Evaluation of Linen service	To review laundry compliance with Australian Standard AS 4146–1994	– AS 4146-1994 – Audit premise practice – Linen care audit	IC Rep, Management & staff	March September	– Compliance with recommended guidelines
Preventative maintenance, bed pan Flusher / Sanitisers	To review compliance with recommended standards AS 2437–1987 and guidelines	– Results of ongoing maintenance from in-house and external contractors	Maintenance	March September	– Ongoing preventative maintenance program – Documentation of routine maintenance

Table 6.1 Lornadoone infection-control quality plan 2003 (cont.)

Activity	Aim of activity	Strategies for implementation & methods used to gain information	Responsibility & liaisons	Target month	Proposed outcome evaluation & intended use of information
Evaluation of staff compliance with Standard Precautions	To assess staff compliance and adherence to NHMRC Guidelines 1998	– Survey check list – Documented guidelines – Observation of staff practice	IC Rep & Management	April	– Staff compliance with recommended guidelines – Implement change as required – Risk control
Evaluation of staff hand washing practices	To assess staff compliance with recommended practice	– Survey check list – Documented guidelines – Observation of staff practice	IC Rep & Management	April January	– Staff compliance with recommended guidelines – Implement change as required – Risk control
Review Environmental Services	To assess compliance between cleaning practices and products used with guidelines.	– Survey of facility – Review of products in use	IC Rep & Management	May	– Techniques for cleaning are those documented

Table 6.1 Lornadoone infection-control quality plan 2003 (cont.)

Evaluation of staff compliance with Standard Precautions	To assess staff compliance and adherence to NHMRC Guidelines 1998	– Staff questionnaire	IC Rep & Management	November / October	– Products used are those that are authorized. – Staff compliance with recommended guidelines – Implement change as required – Risk control
Podiatrists	To assess compliance with Podiatry Association documented guidelines	– DHS documented guidelines – DHS documented guidelines – Podiatry guidelines – NHMRC guidelines	IC Rep & Management	October	– Compliance with recommended guidelines – Risk minimisation
Hairdressers	To assess compliance with DHS documented guidelines	– DHS documented guidelines	IC Rep & Management	November	– Compliance with recommended guidelines – Risk minimisation

Table 6.2 Hand-washing practices audit

(Standard 4—physical environment and safe systems)

Objective: To ensure that staff are aware of appropriate hand washing practices.
Method: Visual observation of staff by infection control committee members on a bi-yearly basis.
Compliance: 100% required.

OBSERVATION	YES	NO	COMMENTS
Are the hands observed for any skin lesions or breaks?			
Is there any nail polish on the fingernails?			
Are the fingernails clean and well maintained?			
Are hands washed under running water?			
Is a soap or antibacterial lotion used?			
Are the hands wet before application of the soap?			
Is jewellery other than a wedding ring worn?			

Table 6.2 Hand-washing practices audit (cont.)

OBSERVATION	YES	NO	COMMENTS
Are all surfaces of the hands, including under the ring, attended to?			
Are the hands washed continuously for 20–30 seconds for a routine hand wash?			
Is a lather created due to friction?			
Are hands rinsed properly?			
Are hands dried properly?			
Is the tap turned off without contamination of the hands?			
Recommendations			

Table 6.3 Linen care audit

(Standard 4—physical environment and safe systems)

Resident care area:

Date:

Observer:

Observed: YES   NO   N/A

Question	Yes	No	N/A
Are gowns worn by staff when making beds or handling linen?			
Is soiled linen carried by staff?			
If soiled linen is carried by staff is it braced against the person's body?			
Is soiled linen placed on the floor?			
Are enough linen skips available in the area?			
Are the linen skips mobile?			
Are the linen skips easily manoeuvred?			
Are linen skips taken to the door of the residents' rooms?			
Are linen skips taken into residents' rooms?			
Is anything draped over the skip to prevent it being moved?			
Are linen skips covered with a drawsheet?			
Does the linen skip have a lid?			
Is the linen skip lid opened by using the foot pedal?			
Is the lid opened by the user's hand?			
Did the user wash hands prior to opening the lid by hand?			
Is the linen pushed down in the skip with the hands?			
Is the staff member observed to wash hands after contact with used linen?			
Are linen bags removed to a storage area when full?			
Are full linen bags dragged across the floor?			

RECOMMENDATIONS:

Table 6.4 Disposal of sharps audit

Objective: To confirm that sharps are disposed of in compliance with EPA
            Guidelines and Australian/New Zealand Standard
            AS/NZS 3816:98 Management of clinical and related waste:

Method: Visual observation of sharps containers and staff practices by infec-
         tion control staff.

Desired Outcome: 100% compliance with documented guidelines required.

Results: YES   NO   N/A

	Site 1	Site 2	Site 3	Site 4	Site 5
Is the sharps container 1.1 to 1.3 metres from the floor?					
Is the sharps container obstructed, requiring staff to reach excessively?					
Are other waste containers placed near sharps containers?					
Is the sharps container greater than 2/3 full?					
Is a lid available on the container?					
Is the lid secured for transport?					
Are full containers secure prior to collection?					
Do the sharps containers contain anything else but sharps?					
Is anything protruding from the opening of the sharps container?					
Are needles and syringes disposed of intact?					
Are the sharps containers shaken to decrease the level of sharps?					
Are staff members observed to wash their hands after contact with sharps?					

RECOMMENDATIONS:

Table 6.5 Single-use items audit

(Standard 4—physical environment and safe systems)

Policy: A single use product is either a product that is used only once and then discarded, or a product that is used by only one resident and then discarded.

Objective: To ensure 100% compliance with the above policy.

Audit Date:

Observer:

OBSERVATION   YES   NO   N/A

Equipment / Supplies	Yes	No	N/A
Syringes			
Needles			
Dressings trays			
Dressings			
Crepe bandages			
Oxygen masks / cannulae			
Nebulisers			
Oxygen Tubing			
Suction catheters			
Indwelling catheter bags			
Makeup			
Combs			
Razors			
Toothbrush			
Toothpaste			
Nail clippers			
Hair rollers			

RESULT: % compliance

RECOMMENDATIONS:

Table 6.6 Staff questionnaires

(Standard 4—physical environment and safe systems)

Objective: To ensure that staff has adequate knowledge regarding infection control practices.
Method: All staff to complete on a yearly basis.
Compliance: 100% required.

Question	TRUE	FALSE
The aim of standard precautions is to reduce cross infection and the risk of acquiring infections between residents and staff.		
All residents blood and body fluids should be treated as if infectious at all times.		
The single most important measure in the prevention of cross infection is hand washing.		
It is necessary to wash your hands after removal of gloves.		
Standard precautions means that protective apparel and practices are utilised when there is a risk of exposure to body substances.		
The principle way that infection is spread is by direct contact.		
Gloves may be reused if they are washed thoroughly.		
Isolation of residents is not required if standard and additional precautions are practiced.		
Hands should be washed after contact with each resident.		
All waste contaminated with blood and body fluids should be placed into a yellow infectious waste bag.		

Table 6.7 Podiatry survey audit

(Standard 4—physical environment and safe systems)

The Podiatrists Registration Board of Victoria requires that all Podiatrists comply with the standards and guidelines; The Infection Control Manual published by the Board, Australian Standard AS 4187-1998 and The NH&MRC guidelines—Infection Control in the Health Care Setting.

Objective: This audit is to assess compliance with the above recommendations when visiting this facility.

Method: All podiatrists attending the facility will be asked to complete this form and practices will be observed by a member of management or the Infection Control representative.

Compliance: 100% required.

Resident care area:

Date:

Observer:

Question	Yes	No
Have you developed any quality activities for your practice?		
Do you regularly complete any quality activities?		
Do you have documented evidence of validation of your sterilising processes?		
Are hands washed prior to resident treatment?		
Is an alcohol based hand rub used for hand hygiene?		
Are gloves worn when there is the potential for contact with body fluids?		
Is a mask worn when there is the potential for contact with body fluids?		
Is protective eyewear worn when there is the potential for contact with body fluids?		
Is a clean, impervious surface used for each resident treatment?		
Are instruments sterile prior to use?		
Are sterile instruments sealed in sterile packaging?		

Table 6.7 Podiatry survey audit (cont.)

Question	Yes	No
Are sterile instruments transported in a clean, sturdy, non porous sealed container		
Are sterile instruments maintained in a clean, dry, dust free environment prior to use?		
Is there a process to ensure that a sterile set of instruments is used for each resident?		
Are gloves removed when interruption to care occurs?		
Are any instruments or equipment, e.g. nail file, used on more than one resident?		
Do all antiseptics remain in their original receptacles?		
Are sterile dressings used as one resident only?		
Are dry, non-sterile, multi use materials stored clean and dry?		
Are sterile and dirty instruments and equipment kept separated?		
Are hands washed on removal of gloves?		
Are hands washed between residents?		
Is cleaning of instruments and equipment attended in a utility room?		
Is a mild alkaline detergent used for cleaning?		
Are any instruments or equipment soaked in antiseptics or disinfectants?		
Are gloves worn when during cleaning procedures?		
Is protective eyewear worn during cleaning procedures?		
Are drill pieces etc cleaned after each resident contact?		
Are storage containers clean and dry?		
Are containers used for sterile items used for any other purpose?		

RECOMMENDATIONS:

Table 6.8 Hairdressing and beauty therapy audit

(Standard 4—physical environment and safe systems)

Objective: This audit is to assess service provider compliance with the Standards of Practice for Hairdressing / Beauty Treatment And Electrolysis, Health (Infectious Diseases) Regulations 1990 when visiting this facility.

Method: All hairdressers/beauticians attending the facility will be asked questions and their practices will be observed by a member of the Infection Control Committee.

Compliance: 100% required.

Date:

Observer:

Question	Yes	No	Comments / Examples
Have you submitted a copy of your Certificate of Registration Health Act (1958) as a mobile hairdresser from local government authority?			
Have you submitted a photocopy of your graduation certificate or trade certificate from the Sate training Board of Victoria?			
Have you submitted a copy of your registration of Company or Business?			
Have you submitted identification to verify your name?			
Have you confirmed that you have adequate Public Liability Insurance?			
Do you check in at reception on your arrival at the facility?			
Have you developed any quality activities for your practice if so, what?			
Is the operator well groomed?			
Do you check your hands for any cuts, lesions or abrasions before commencing service?			

Table 6.8 Hairdressing and beauty therapy audit (cont.)

Question	Yes	No	Comments / Examples
If any cuts, lesions or abrasions are present is the area covered with an occlusive dressing and plastic gloves worn?			
Does the equipment to be used appear to be clean?			
Are hands washed prior to resident treatment?			
Is an alcohol based hand rub used for hand hygiene?			
Are articles and equipment cleaned between clients?			
Is the residents skin (scalp) checked prior to commencement of service?			
Are single use disposable razors or blades used?			
Are single use disposable razors or blades disposed of into sharps containers?			
Are hands washed between residents?			
Are neck brushes used, if so how are they cleaned?			
Are instruments and equipment washed / rinsed with hot water not less than 70degrees C?			
Are any disinfectants used to decontaminate articles or equipment?			
Are any instruments or equipment, eg nail file, used on more than one resident?			

Table 6.8 Hairdressing and beauty therapy audit (cont.)

Question	Yes	No	Comments / Examples
Are containers of creams or ointments contaminated after use?			
Are instruments and equipment that cannot be washed/rinsed with hot water wiped with 70% alcohol?			
Are towels, wraps and other washable fabric washed with hot water not less than 70degrees C?			
What do you do if scissors or other sharp instruments accidentally cut a resident?			

RECOMMENDATIONS:

Table 6.9 Cleaning audit

(Standard 4—physical environment and safe systems)

Policy: The facility and environment is to be maintained in a clean state free from dust, dirt and any soiling.

Objective: To assess compliance with documented policy and schedules.

Audit Date: Observer: Area:

Criteria	Acceptable		Action Required
	Yes	No	
Is the environment aesthetically pleasing?			
Are doors and door handles free from fingermarks and residual soil?			
Are windows clean inside and out?			
Do curtains show any signs of soiling?			
Is there any dust on curtain tracks, windowsills or door jams?			
Are light fittings clean with no insects or dust inside fitting?			
Are bedside tables and overbed tables clean and free from marks and food residue?			
Is the bed linen clean?			
Is all furniture clean and free from dust?			
Is the wardrobe tidy with a clean floor?			
Is all equipment clean and free from residual soilage?			
Are all personal belongings clean and dust free?			
Is the carpet clean and free from residual dirt (including under furniture) and odours?			
Are hard floors free from dust and scuff marks?			
Are skirting boards and window ledges clean?			
Are air vents clean with no dust?			
Is the waste bin clean, have a liner and no odours or residual soiling?			
Other			

Result: % compliance

Table 6.10 Storage of sterile stock audit

Aim: To review the transport and storage of sterile stock across.

Objective: To assess compliance with Australian / New Zealand Standard AS/NZS 4187 / 2003.

Method: Observation by an experienced person e.g. an infection control CNC and / or the nurse unit manager.

Site: Date:

Transport

Issue	Yes	No	Comments
Is all sterile stock handled with care by delivery staff?			
Are the trolleys used to transport sterile stock clean?			
Is sterile stock delivered in the appropriate containers?			
Is sterile stock placed on the floor on delivery?			

Storage

Issue	Yes	No	Comments
Is sterile stock stored away immediately after delivery?			
Is sterile stock confined to a dedicated area within the facility?			
Is there any sterile stock stored outside the dedicated area?			
Is stock removed from outer packaging / boxes?			
Is there unnecessary handling of packaged goods causing compromise to the packaging? i.e. separating needles.			

Table 6.10 Storage of sterile stock audit (cont.)

Issue	Yes	No	Comments
Does there appear to be overstocking?			
Does there appear to be mixing of batch numbers?			
Are all items > 250mm above the floor?			
Are all items > 400mm from ceiling fixtures?			
Is all sterile stock protected from natural sunlight?			
Is the storage area part of a public thoroughfare?			
Are any procedures attended in close proximity to sterile stock storage?			
Is the storage area clean and dust free?			
Are rubber bands used to contain packaged items?			
Are there any areas difficult to clean?			
Are storage containers maintained in good condition?			
Are storage containers clean and dry?			
Are storage containers regularly cleaned?			

Recommendation:

Table 6.11 An example of a completed quality-assurance activity report of linen care using the linen-care audit table

Audit: Linen care			Standard: 4.7—Linen care	
Plan			Progress report	
Aim/s of activity	Methodology		Data analysis (results)	Actions taken/evaluation
To assess compliance with recommended and documented guidelines.	Observing staff members handling soiled and clean linen.		Six staff members were observed.	Facility guidelines were reviewed.
	Guidelines used: • Infection control manual • Australian Standard AS 4146 2000.		Overall, there was 75% compliance with the recommended guidelines. Concerns: • Soiled linen carried by staff. • Skips taken to the door. • Skips not taken in to rooms. • Hands not washed after contact with used linen.	Representatives of the Infection Control Committee re-educated staff. Regular inservice education planned.

Date: April 2003

Signature

Table 6.12 Infection-control worksheet

INFECTION CONTROL WORKSHEET

Name of facility   Month   Year

Number	Staff/ resident's name	Infection site	Date infection identified	Pathology tests		Interventions		Health & nutritional status	Possible cause			
				Site	Organism identified	Antibiotics	Nursing		Nursing practice	Procedure/ policy	Equipment/ environment	Other

Print name

Signature

© Kevin Kendall

Table 6.13 Infection-control monthly statistics

INFECTION CONTROL MONTHLY STATISTICS					
Name of Facility			Month	Year	
Infection sites	Number of Infections due to identified causative factors				
	Resident health/nutritional status	Nursing practices	Policy/procedure non-compliance	Equipment/ environment	Other
Skin and mucous membrane					
Urinary tract					
Respiratory tract: ear, nose, throat and mouth					
Eye					
Systemic					
Skeletal and connective tissue					

© Kevin Kendall

Table 6.14 Infection-control action sheet

Name of facility		Month		Year	
INFECTION CONTROL ACTION SHEET					
Issue	Action frame	Time frame	Person responsible	Results	Recommendations	Date, sign and print name

© Kevin Kendall

Table 6.15 Infection-control yearly statistics

Name of Facility													Year		
Site of infection	*Causative factors	MONTH													
		Jan	Feb	Mar	Apr	May	Jun	Jul	Aug	Sept	Oct	Nov	Dec
Skin and mucous membrane	R												
	N												
	P												
	E												
	O												
Urinary tract	R												
	N												
	P												
	E												
	O												
Respiratory tract: ear, nose, throat and mouth	R												
	N												
	P												
	E												
	O												
Eye	R												
	N												
	P												
	E												
	O												
Systemic	R												
	N												
	P												
	E												
	O												
Skeletal and connective tissue	R												
	N												
	P												
	E												
	O												

* Causative factors key: R=resident; N=nursing; P=policy or procedure; E=equipment; O=other

(from Infection Control Worksheet)

Classification of infections

In order to collect data that can be analysed, the types of infections reported during the month must be classified in a meaningful way. The following classification of infections is not meant to be definitive. Rather, it is a general practical guideline, derived from international standards to assist data collectors in deciding which indicators of infection should be included in a local audit.

Definitions

The following definitions are adapted from McGeer et al. (1991).[9] They are based on three important principles:

- symptoms of infection must be new or acutely worse—i.e., there is a change in an individual's status;
- non-infectious causes must be eliminated before infection is diagnosed;
- the clinical picture, microbiology, and radiological findings should all be considered when making a diagnosis.

Respiratory tract infections

Common cold

At least two of the following must be present:

- runny nose, sneezing;
- congestion;
- sore throat, hoarseness, or difficulty swallowing;
- dry cough;
- cervical lymphadenopathy;
- fever (might or may not be present).

Influenza-like illnesses

The following must be present for a diagnosis of influenza to be made:

- fever of 38°C (temperature can be recorded from any body site);
- at least three of the following: chills, new headache, eye pain, myalgia, malaise, reduced appetite, sore throat, new cough, exacerbated dry cough.

In cases in which the influenza-like illness coincides with another respiratory tract infection, influenza should be the primary diagnosis.

Pneumonia

The person must have a chest X-ray consistent with pneumonia and new infiltrate must be present compared with previous chest X-rays.

In addition, at least two of the following should be present:

- new or increased cough and/or sputum production;
- fever 38°C;
- pleuritic chest pain;
- new or increased rhonchi, wheeze, or bronchial breathing.
- difficulty breathing;
- new or increased shortness of breath or respiratory rate of at least 25 breaths per minute;
- significant deterioration in cognitive status and/or self-care ability.

Bronchitis, tracheobronchitis

At least three of signs and symptoms described for pneumonia must be present.

Urinary tract infections

Only symptomatic urinary tract infections (UTIs) are included because many residents have asymptomatic UTIs.

No indwelling catheter

Three of the following must be present:

- fever 38°C;
- chills;
- burning pain on mictuition;
- frequency or urgency;
- flank or suprapubic tenderness;
- change in character of the urine (e.g., blood or pus, changed cognitive and self-care capacity).

Indwelling catheter in place

At least two of the above symptoms (although changes associated with mictuition will not be present). Urine cultures might not be helpful if the patient is on antibiotics.

Conjunctivitis

One of the following symptoms is diagnostic:

- pus from one or both eyes that has been present for at least 24 hours;
- new or increased conjunctival redness for at least 24 hours.

Note that pain might or may not be present. Allergy and trauma must be excluded.

Ear infections

New discharge from one or both ears. If the discharge is not purulent other signs of inflammation must be present. Ear infections are diagnosed by a doctor.

Oral infections

These include candidiasis. They must be diagnosed by a doctor.

Cellulitis

Signs and symptoms include:

- redness, pain, or swelling;
- pus from a wound, skin or soft tissue;
- fever 38°C;
- worsening cognitive or self-care status.

Fungal skin infection

The resident must have skin evidence of an infection (e.g, a rash). The diagnosis is made by a doctor and/or a laboratory diagnosis.

Herpes (simplex or zoster)

Vesicular rash and laboratory or doctor diagnosis.

Scabies

A maculopapular rash and itching. Diagnosis is made by a doctor and/or laboratory. Allergy and secondary skin irritation must be excluded.

Gastrointestinal tract infection

At least one of the following criteria must be met in a 24-hour period:

- watery stools that are different from normal;
- two episodes of vomiting together with diarrhoea, abdominal pain. positive stool culture for pathogenic organism, positive toxin assay.

Medications and other causes of gastrointestinal symptoms must be excluded.

Systemic infection

Primary septicaemia can be diagnosed in the presence of one of the following:

- two blood cultures positive for the same organism;
- a single positive blood culture not caused by a contaminant *and* at least one of the following—fever of 38°C; new hypothermia (34.5°C or not registering); drop in systolic blood pressure of 30 mm Hg; deteriorating cognitive or functional status.

Chapter 7

Common Infections and

Infectious Diseases

Introduction

This chapter discusses some of the important features of common infections and infectious diseases.[1, 2, 3]

The common cold

The common cold (*coryza*), is usually a mild viral illness. However, it does cause disruption to work routines and can lead to complications in vulnerable people. It has an incubation period of 2–3 days, and the infectious period is present while the affected individual is coughing and sneezing.

Controlling the spread of the common cold involves:

- covering mouth and nose when coughing and sneezing;
- careful disposal of used tissues; and
- restricting contact with others.

Treatment usually consists of symptomatic treatment (such as paracetamol-containing medicines and decongestants). Antibiotics are inappropriate unless there are bacterial complications.

Influenza

Influenza is an acute viral illness of the respiratory tract caused by a virus. Signs and symptoms last from 2–7 days and can include:

- fever and chills;
- headache and muscle pain;
- a head cold and mild sore throat; and
- severe cough.

The incubation period lasts 1–5 days, and the affected person is infectious for three days from the onset of signs and symptoms.

Controlling the spread of influenza involves staff members not attending for work, and the segregation of affected residents from other residents until the symptoms subside.

Usually only symptomatic treatment (such as paracetamol-containing medicines and decongestants) is required. Antibiotics are given only for bacterial complications.

Prevention is important and annual autumn influenza vaccination is recommended in the following groups of people:

- those with chronic debilitating illnesses (such as asthma, diabetes, or heart disease);
- those over 65 years of age;
- those receiving immunosuppressive therapy; and
- those who work in medical and health services.

Chickenpox

Chickenpox is a highly contagious viral illness with the following signs and symptoms:

- a cough and runny nose (similar to a common cold);
- fever and tiredness; followed by
- a generalised rash.

The rash begins as raised bumps that develop into sores with blister-like heads. After three or four days the sores crust over. However, there can be several crops of blisters and sores at various stages of development. The rash can occur anywhere on the body but is usually more noticeable on the trunk.

One episode of infection generally gives immunity from further attacks of chickenpox. Second infections are rare, but the virus can remain dormant in the nerve cells for the rest of a person's life.

The incubation period usually lasts for 2–3 weeks (commonly 13–17 days). The affected person remains infectious from two days before the rash appears, during the coughing and runny nose stage, and until all blisters have crusted over.

Chickenpox is spread by coughing and direct contact with the blister fluid. The spread of the disease is controlled as follows.

- People who have not had chickenpox should not care for people with chickenpox.
- Segregate people with chickenpox until all blisters have crusted over (no moist sores) and the person feels well.
- Carefully dispose of tissues soiled with nose and throat discharge.
- Wash hands after contact with soiled articles.
- Ensure that good cleaning procedures are followed (especially if articles have been soiled with nose and throat discharge).

Symptomatic treatment is usually all that is required—for example, topical applications for itching.

Herpes zoster (shingles)

Herpes zoster occurs when the chickenpox virus in the body becomes activated after being dormant for a period of time. Skin eruptions occur with blisters that form sores on well-defined areas of the body, usually in the area of the nerve where the virus has lain dormant. Shingles is often associated with severe pain that can last for some time.

Direct contact with the moist shingles rash can cause chickenpox in a person who has never had chickenpox.

Infection control consists of the following measures.

- People who have not had chickenpox should not care for people with shingles.
- Avoid exposure to the moist shingles blisters.
- Zoster immunoglobin (ZIG) can be considered for contacts at very high risk of complications because of other medical problems.
- Wash hands after contact with soiled articles.
- Ensure good cleaning procedures are followed.
- Symptomatic treatment (such as pain relief) is the usual treatment.

Herpes simplex Type 1 (cold sores)

Herpes simplex occurs as single or multiple lesions—most commonly in or near the mouth (at the junction of skin and mucous membranes. However, it can occur in other body areas—such as the gums, mouth, eyes, and labia.

Signs and symptoms include redness, tingling, and the appearance of blisters.

Once a person is infected, the virus remains dormant, but it can recur at any time— triggered by illness, stress, sunlight, or hormonal changes. The incubation period is usually between 2 and 12 days, and the person remains infectious until the infected area has completely dried.

Control of spread involves the following measures.

- Isolation is unnecessary, but hand-washing and cleaning procedures must be strictly observed.
- Avoid kissing on or near the infected area.
- Do not share food or drink containers.
- Dispose of used tissues carefully and immediately.
- Staff with lesions on their fingers should not attend for work until the lesions are dry.
- If lesions are present on the hands, they must be washed frequently and kept away from the face.

Treatment consists of antiviral medication (such as oral and topical acyclovir) commenced at the first symptoms of an herpetic eruption—often a tingling sensation.

Conjunctivitis

The term 'conjunctivitis' refers to an irritation or infection of the eye caused by bacteria, viruses, chemicals, or allergies. The diagnosis can be aided by microscopy and culture of a swab.

Signs and symptoms can include:

- redness;
- discharge;
- itching, scratchy feeling;
- stickiness; and
- sensitivity to light.

Conjunctivitis is spread directly by contact with eye secretions, or indirectly by contaminated face washers, towels, handkerchiefs, or eye drops.

The incubation period is 24–72 hours, and the affected person is infectious during the course of the active bacterial or viral infection, or until three days after beginning antibiotic treatment for a bacterial infection. Conjunctivitis caused by chemicals or allergies is not infectious.

Control of spread involves the following measures.

- Discourage contact with other people during the infectious stage.
- Good personal hygiene—such as careful hand washing using soap and warm water.
- Avoid sharing towels and washcloths.
- Eye drops must never be shared.
- Dispose of eye drops after the prescribed course is completed.

Treatment consists of antibiotic eye drops or ointments prescribed by a doctor. The treatment should be continued until the full prescribed course has been completed. The drops or ointment should be instilled after a careful eye toilet.

Gastroenteritis

There are many varieties of gastroenteritis. Spread is by the faecal–oral route. The incubation period is variable—depending on the causative organism. The infectious period also depends on the causative organism. However, in general, precautions should be taken for up to a week after the last episode of vomiting or diarrhoea.

Control of spread involves the following measures.
- good personal hygiene;
- careful hand washing;
- segregation of infected people;
- careful disposal of the vomit and faeces from an infected person;
- adequate washing of the utensils, crockery and cutlery used by an infected person;
- exclusion of infected staff from work until asymptomatic;
- good housekeeping practices (e.g., cleaning);

Clusters of infected people should be reported to the health department.

Treatment is symptomatic, including fluid replacement. Extreme care must be taken with affected elderly people because dehydration can have a devastating effect.

If the illness is severe it is essential to maintain fluid balance, provide electrolyte replacement as indicated, and administer prescribed antidiarrhoeal and antiemetic medications.

Laboratory investigation are essential to establish the causative organism. Antibiotic therapy has a limited role in some types of gastroenteritis.

Prevention involves the following:
- storing foods carefully, and transporting and handling food correctly;
- eating only well-cooked meat;
- careful hand washing;
- careful washing of fruit and vegetables before consumption; and
- controlling pests and vermin.

Meningitis

Meningitis can be caused by a variety of viruses and bacteria. Some bacterial forms of meningitis can be rapidly fatal unless promptly diagnosed and treated. Meningitis can occur in epidemics, with a number of infected people presenting with fever, headache, rash, and joint pains. Severe headache, neck stiffness, and intolerance of light (photophobia) are common features of all forms of the disease. Irritability might be the only early sign in elderly people.

The incubation period varies from hours to days, depending on the infecting organism. The infectious period is present from just before and during the acute phase of the illness.

Control of spread involves the following measures:

- covering the mouth and nose when coughing and sneezing;
- good personal hygiene;
- hand washing;
- staff wearing protective apparel;
- proper disposal of waste;
- public health measures (such as following up people who have been in contact with an infected person); and
- affected people completing the prescribed course of antibiotic therapy.

Treatment involves the following:

- laboratory investigation to establish the causative organism;
- symptomatic treatment (such as analgesics and antiemetics);
- specific antibiotic therapy (for bacterial menignitis);
- supportive care (such as hospitalisation for rehydration).

Prevention involves:

- prophylactic antibiotic therapy for family members and contacts (if appropriate);
- recommended vaccination for children;
- control of pests and vermin; and
- preventing inhalation of dust.

Hepatitis

Hepatitis is inflammation of the liver caused by bacteria, viruses, medication, alcohol, or non-prescribed, so-called 'recreational' drugs. The condition can vary in severity. Jaundice, nausea and vomiting, and dark urine and pale faeces can be present.

There are several varieties of hepatitis. The most prevalent varieties in developed countries are hepatitis A, hepatitis B, and hepatitis C. Hepatitis E is a major cause of waterborne epidemics in developing countries.

Hepatitis A

Signs and symptoms of hepatitis A can last from a few weeks to several months. Young children can have the disease with no apparent signs or symptoms. There is no treatment for hepatitis A once symptoms develop.

Signs and symptoms of hepatitis A include:

- abdominal tenderness;
- fever;

- nausea;
- tiredness;
- jaundice—yellowing of the skin and whites of the eyes; and
- pale faeces and dark urine.

The incubation period lasts 15–50 days (usually 28–30 days). A person is most infectious in the two weeks before jaundice occurs, and slightly infectious during the first week of jaundice.

Control of spread involves the following measures:

- isolation of the person for one week after the onset of jaundice or illness;
- all people who come in to contact with the infected person should be offered immunoglobulin which, if given within two weeks of exposure, usually prevents hepatitis A, or causes its signs and symptoms to be milder;
- staff must practise careful hand washing and cleaning procedures;
- do not share towels.

Hepatitis B

Hepatitis B is a mild to severe viral infection of the liver that can cause jaundice. The majority of adults who are infected do not suffer a serious illness and do not develop jaundice. However, a few people who contract hepatitis B become long-term carriers of the disease. There is a risk of liver cirrhosis and liver cancer for long-term carriers. There is no specific treatment for hepatitis B, other than rest.

Hepatitis B is a human viral infection, and is not found in animals. Most Australians are not at significant risk of exposure to hepatitis B. However, some groups in the community can have a higher risk of exposure—due to their background, lifestyle, or occupation. High-risk groups include:

- Asian migrants;
- indigenous Australians;
- intravenous drug users; and
- those occupationally at risk of blood-to-blood exposure (e.g., nurses, personal carers, doctors, dentists, and laboratory workers).

All people participating in high-risk activities should be immunised against hepatitis B. Transmission is through unprotected sexual intercourse and blood-to-blood contact (such as when intravenous drug users share needles).

The incubation period lasts between 45 and 180 days, with an average of 60–90 days. The infectious period occurs from one month before jaundice to 1–3 months after jaundice appears. Some people can carry the virus for life.

Control of spread involves the following measures.

- Carriers should be educated about the risks of transmitting the disease. It is not necessary to isolate carriers or those who have active disease.
- Staff must observe standard precautions when handling any blood-contaminated items.
- Blood and body fluid spills must be dealt with effectively.
- Staff must practise careful hand-washing.
- Routinely cover open sores, cuts, and abrasions.
- Immunisation should be available for those in high-risk situations.
- Following accidental exposure to hepatitis B (e.g., a puncture wound from an infected needle), hepatitis B immunoglobulin (HBIG) should be given immediately. It is available from the Red Cross Transfusion Service.

Hepatitis C

Hepatitis C, a bloodborne viral infection, can result in an illness similar to hepatitis B. Hepatitis C was first recognised in 1989. At that time approximately 40% of people acquired hepatitis C via blood transfusions, 40% by sharing needles, and the remainder from unidentified sources. Since then, Australian blood supplies have been screened to reduce the risk of acquiring hepatitis C from blood products. It is not clear if hepatitis C can be transmitted sexually.

The incubation period is from 2 to 6 months (usually 6–9 weeks). The infectious period lasts from one or two weeks before the first symptoms (acute stage), but can last indefinitely (chronic carrier stage).

A person with hepatitis C need not be isolated. Because hepatitis C is a bloodborne virus, control strategies include educating those infected about the risks of needle-stick injury and unsafe sexual practices.

There is no specific treatment for hepatitis C, other than rest.

Legionnaires' disease

Legionnaires' disease results from infection by the Legionella group of bacteria—usually causing a form of pneumonia. However, Legionella can sometimes cause 'Pontiac fever'—a 'flu-like illness that does not involve the lungs.

The signs and symptoms of Legionnaires' disease include severe fever, sweating, headaches, and muscular aches and pains. Infection without symptoms is common.

Legionella organisms thrive in moist areas such as:

- hot-water systems and air-conditioning cooling towers;
- hot and cold water taps;
- showers;
- garden soil or potting mix.

The bacteria must be inhaled to cause disease. Legionnaires' disease occurs most commonly in the warmer months. Predisposing factors include:

- age;
- cigarette smoking;
- heavy alcohol use;
- other illness; and
- stress.

The incubation period is from two to ten days (usually five to six days). Transmission from person-to-person has not been documented.

Prevention involves the following measures.

- Cooling towers should be drained when not in use, cleaned periodically to remove scale and sediment, and maintained according to Guidelines 4.
- Appropriate chemicals should be used to limit the growth of slime-forming organisms in any water-processing system.
- Showers can be tested after maintenance.
- Careful hand-washing must be practised after contact with garden soil or potting mix.

Treatment consists of specific antibiotic treatment, commenced once the diagnosis is made. Severe cases need hospital care, which might involve intensive care.

Scabies and other skin disease-causing mites

Scabies mites infest the skin between the fingers, on the wrists, and in the skin folds of the body. Thread-like 'tunnels', approximately 10 mm long, give the appearance of dark dots on the infected skin—but these are often difficult to identify. Skin disease caused by scabies and other mites is diagnosed by microscopic examination of skin scrapings.

Scabies and other mites usually cause itching which varies from slight to intense. It is more of a problem at night than during the day. Hot showers and baths stimulate further itching and scratching, and this can lead to secondary infection.

Transmission is usually by skin-to-skin contact, but the organisms can be transferred from clothing or bedclothes that have been freshly contaminated by an infested person. The mites survive for only a few days off the human or animal body. Scabies mites from animals can live on humans, but do not reproduce in the skin.

Some forms of skin disease in animals caused by mites can also spread to humans. If an animal has mange, it is important to have a veterinarian diagnose which mite is causing the mange—because some animal mange mites spread to humans.

Itching from mite infestation begins 2–6 weeks after the first infestation in first-time infections. However, previously exposed and reinfested individuals start scratching within 1–4 days. People remain contagious until the mites and eggs are destroyed by treatment.

Control of spread involves the following measures.

- Segregate people with mites until the day after treatment.
- Wash all clothing and bed linen.
- Items that cannot be washed should be dry cleaned or placed in a sealed garbage bag for seven days, then aired before use.
- Close contacts should be inspected for signs of infestation.

Treatment involves the following:

- Initial treatment with solutions such as Lindane or Quellada (with repeat treatment in seven days).
- Attention must be paid to under the fingernails.
- Antihistamines might be required to control the itch (which can persist for up two weeks after successful treatment).
- In cases of proven or strongly suspected treatment failure, a treatment with permethrin (Lyclear) is recommended.
- Repeated treatment with Quellada should be avoided.

Tuberculosis

Tuberculosis (TB) is mainly a bacterial infection of the lungs, but it can affect other parts of the body (such as kidneys or bone). The bacteria are transmitted by droplets from people with active disease. These are spread during coughing, sneezing, singing, or talking. Few infected children have signs or symptoms.

After infecting a host, the tubercule organism can lie dormant for many years. However, whether the disease is active or not, it takes only 4–12 weeks from infection for a positive skin test to develop. The risk of active disease is greatest within the first two years of infection.

Young children rarely transmit the disease, even if they have a positive skin test. However, adults are infectious as long as they have active TB and are not under treatment.

Control of spread involves the following measures.

- If a person is found to have active TB, he or she should be segregated until 10 days after appropriate treatment has been commenced.
- Sputum must be disposed of carefully.
- People who have been in contact with the infected person can be skin tested.

Treatment is required for active TB and people must receive medication under the supervision of a doctor and/or a state government tuberculosis unit.

HIV and AIDS

The effect of infection with the human immune-deficiency virus (HIV) varies. A person with the virus—as indicated by a positive antibody test—can have no immediate apparent disease. However, weight loss, diarrhoea, and malaise can develop. The fully developed disease—acquired immune deficiency syndrome (AIDS) is characterised by repeated infections with unusual organisms that do not affect people with healthy immune systems. People with AIDS are also at risk of developing unusual cancers.

Transmission is by:

- skin penetration by infected blood (for example, from accidental occupational exposure through a needle-stick injury, or from sharing infected needles and syringes when injecting drugs);
- transfusion with infected blood products;
- sexual intercourse (anal, oral, or vaginal) with an infected person; or
- infected mother-to-child (before or during birth, or via breast milk).

HIV is not transmitted by:

- ordinary social contact in schools, at home, or in the workplace;
- air or water;
- sharing plates, cups, cutlery;

- community swimming pools or toilets;
- kissing people with active disease;
- singing, coughing, sneezing, or spitting; or
- the bites of mosquitoes or other insects.

The effects of infection might not be evident for months or years after HIV infection. In about 70% of infected adults, a glandular fever-like illness occurs about one month after infection. This is known as seroconversion. AIDS develops within ten years of infection in at least 50% of HIV-infected people. New treatments are lowering this rate.

The infectious period exists from two to four weeks after infection with the virus. However, because it takes three months before antibodies are produced, a blood test (positive or negative) actually indicates the HIV status *as it was* three months before the blood was taken. This is called the 'window period'. Some people test positive to the virus but remain well. However, it seems likely that HIV infection is lifelong and that infected people will always remain potentially infectious.

Only people who come into physical contact with human blood, body tissue, and secretions are at risk of acquiring HIV infection through occupational exposure. Care should be taken when exposure to body fluids or blood of any type occurs. The risk of occupational exposure can be minimised if infection-control guidelines (as outlined in the Worksafe Australia publication 'HIV and the Workplace: Information for Health Workers and Others at Risk[5]) are followed. In brief, policies to prevent the workplace transmission of HIV should aim to:

- reassure workers that the risk of transmission of HIV is minimal with safe work practices;
- protect workers and the general public from exposure; and
- maintain full civil and industrial rights for infected workers (i.e., ensure confidentiality and that HIV positive staff are not discriminated against).

There is no need to segregate items such as eating utensils, plates, and cups. The usual cleaning techniques are sufficient for toilets and washing facilities. In the rare instance of a staff member being required to perform resuscitation on a person who is infected with HIV, simple precautions should be taken—including the use of mechanical ventilators and disposable or sterilisable mouth-to-mouth masks. The risk during direct mouth-to-mouth contact is extremely low, and resuscitation should never be withheld. All facilities should ensure that staff members have been educated to supply emergency treatment without putting themselves at risk.

Appendices

Appendix A
Australian and New Zealand health departments

Australian Capital Territory

Australian Capital Territory Health
GPO Box 825
Canberra City 2601
Australian Capital Territory
Telephone: (02) 6207 5111

New South Wales

Health Department
Locked Mail Bag 961
North Sydney 2059
New South Wales
Telephone: (02) 9391 9000

Northern Territory

Department of Health & Community
  Services
PO Box 40596
Casuarina 0811
Northern Territory
Telephone: (08) 8999 2400

New Zealand

New Zealand Health Service
PO Box 5013
Wellington
New Zealand
Telephone: 644 922 1800

Queensland

Department of Health
GPO Box 48
Brisbane 4001
Queensland
Telephone: (07) 3234 0111

South Australia

Department of Human Services & Public
  Health
PO Box 6
Rundle Mall
Adelaide 5000
South Australia
Telephone: (08) 8226 7107

Tasmania

Department of Human Services
GPO Box 125
Hobart 7001
Tasmania
(03) 6233 3185

Victoria

Department of Human Services
555 Collins St
Melbourne 3000
Victoria
Telephone: (03) 9616 7777 or
1300 651 160

Western Australia

Health Department of Western Australia
PO Box 8172
Perth Business Centre
Perth 6849
Western Australia
Telephone: 1300 135 030

Appendix B

The following pages contain a list of infectious diseases currently notifiable in Australia, presented state-by-state and in New Zealand. Notifiable infectious diseases are reviewed on a regular basis, and diseases are added to or removed from the list according to the relevant health department's decisions. To obtain up-to-date information, contact the relevant health department. Contact details can be found in Appendix A.

Australian Capital Territory

Anthrax
Acquired immune deficiency syndrome
  (AIDS)
Arbovirus infection
Botulism
Brucellosis
Campylobacteriosis
Chlamydial disease
Cholera
Dengue
Diphtheria
Donovanosis (granuloma inguinale)
Food poisoning
Gonorrhoea
Haemophilus influenzae type B infection
Hepatitis (viral)
Hepatitis A
Hepatitis B
Hepatitis C
Human immune deficiency virus (HIV)
  infection
Hydatid infection
Legionellosis
Leprosy
Leptospirosis
Listeriosis
Lymphogranuloma venereum
Malaria
Measles
Meningococcal infection
Mumps
Pertussis
Plague
Poliomyelitis
Psittacosis and other forms of ornithosis
Q fever
Rabies
Ross River virus infection
Rubella
Salmonellosis
Shigellosis
Syphilis
Tetanus
Tuberculosis
Typhoid and paratyphoid

Viral haemorrhagic fever
Yellow Fever
Yersiniosis

New South Wales

AIDS
Anthrax
Adverse event following immunisation
Arbovirus infection (Flavivirus)
Botulism
Brucellosis
Chancroid
Cholera
Cryptosporidiosis
Diphtheria
Foodborne illness in two or more related
  cases
Gastroenteritis (among persons in an
  institution)
Giardiasis
Gonorrhoea
Haemolytic uraemic syndrome
Haemophilus influenzae type B invasive
Hepatitis A
Hepatitis B
Hepatitis C
Hepatitis D
Hepatitis E
HIV
Legionella infections
Legionnaires' disease
Leprosy
Leptospirosis
Listeriosis
Lymphogranuloma venerum
Lyssavirus
Malaria
Measles
Meningococcal disease

Mumps
Mycobacterial disease
Paratyphoid
Pertussis (whooping cough)
Plague
Pneumococcal invasive infection
Poliomyelitis
Psittacosis
Q fever
Rabies
Rubella (German measles)
Salmonella infections
Shigellosis
Syphilis
Tetanus
Tuberculosis
Typhoid
Typhus (epidemic)
Verotoxin-producing *Escherichia coli*
  infections
Viral haemorrhagic fevers
Yellow fever

New Zealand

AIDS
Acute gastroenteritis
Anthrax
Arbovirus diseases
Brucellosis
Campylobacteriosis
Cholera
Creutzfeldt Jakob disease and other
  spongiform
Encephalopathies
Cryptosporidiosis
Cysticercosis
Diphtheria
Giardiasis
Haemophilus influenzae B
Hepatitis (viral)
Hepatitis A

Hepatitis B
Hepatitis C
Hydatid disease
Legionellosis
Leprosy
Leptospirosis
Listeriosis
Malaria
Measles
Meningoencephalitis—primary amoebic
Mumps
Pertussis
Plague
Poliomyelitis
Rabies
Rheumatic fever
Rickettsial diseases
Rubella
Salmonellosis
Shigellosis
Tetanus
Trichinosis
Tuberculosis
Typhoid and paratyphoid fever
Viral haemorrhagic fevers
Yellow fever
Yersiniosis

Northern Territory

Acute post-streptococcal glomerulonephritis
Adverse vaccine reactions
AIDS
Amoebiasis
Anthrax
Arbovirus infection
Australian Encephalitis (MVE, Kunjin):
• Bumah Forest virus
• Dengue

• River virus
• Non-specified
Atypical mycobacterium
Botulism (foodborne)
Brucellosis
Campylobactoriosis
Chancroid
Chlamydia infection
Cholera
Congenital rubella
Congenital syphilis
Diphtheria
Donovanosis (Granuloma inguinale)
Ebola virus disease
Gonococcal infection
Haemophilus influenzae type B
Hepatitis A
Hepatitis B
Hepatitis C
Hepatitis D
Hepatitis E
HIV
Hydatid infection
Lassa fever
Legionellosis
Leprosy (Hansen's disease)
Leptospirosis
Listeriosis
Lymphogranuloma venereum
Malaria
Marburg virus disease
Measles
Meningococcal infection
Mumps
Pertussis
Plague
Pneumococcal disease (invasive)
Poliomyelitis
Q Fever
Rabies

Rheumatic fever
Rotavirus infection
Rubella
Salmonellosis
Shigellosis
Smallpox
Syphilis
Tetanus
Tuberculosis
Typhoid & paratyphoid
Typhus (all forms)
Viral haemorrhagic fever
Yellow fever
Yersiniosis

Queensland

Acute viral hepatitis
Adverse event following vaccination
Anthrax
Arbovirus infections (specified)
Atypical mycobacterial infection
Botulism
Brucellosis
Carnpylobacter enteritis
Chancroid
Chlamydia trachomatis infections
Cholera
Cryptococcosis
Cryptosporidiosis
Diphtheria
Donovanosis (granuloma inguinale)
Echinococcosis (hydatid disease)
Enterohaemorrhagic Escherichia coli
   infection
Equine morbilli virus infection
Food-borne or water-borne illness in two
   or more associated cases
Gonococcal infection
Haemolytic uraemic syndrome

Haemophilus influenzae type B infection
Hansen's disease (leprosy)
Hepatitis A
Hepatitis B
Hepatitis C
Hepatitis D
Hepatitis E
HIV
Legionellosis
Leptospirosis
Listeriosis
Lymphogranuloma venereum
Malaria
Marburg viruses
Measles
Meningococcal infection (invasive)
Mumps
Pertussis
Plague
Pneumococcal disease (invasive)
Poliomyelitis
Q fever
Rabies
Rubella
Salmonellosis
Shigellosis
Syphilis
Tetanus
Tuberculosis
Typhoid and paratyphoid
Viral haemorrhagic fevers (Crimean-
   Congo, Ebola, Lassa fever and
   yersiniosis)

South Australia

AIDS
Arbovirus infection
Atypical mycobacterial infection
Barmah Forest virus

Botulism
Brucellosis
Campylobacter infection
Chlamydia infection (genital)
Cholera
Congenital rubella syndrome
Cryptosporidiosis
Dengue fever
Diphtheria
Food poisoning (two or more related
  cases)
Gonococcal infection
Haemophilus influenzae infection
Hepatitis A
Hepatitis B
HIV infection
Hydatid disease
Legionellosis
Leprosy
Leptospirosis
Listeriosis
Malaria
Measles
Meningococcal infection
Mumps
Murray Valley encephalitis virus
Ornithosis (psittacosis)
Paratyphoid infection
Pertussis (whooping cough)
Plague
Poliomyelitis
Psittacosis
Q fever
Rabies (human)
Ross River virus
Rubella
Salmonella infection
Shigella infection
Syphilis
Tetanus
Tuberculosis

Typhoid infection
Viral haemorrhagic fevers
Whooping cough
Yellow fever
Yersinia infection

Tasmania
Amoebiasis
Anthrax
Arbovirus infection (including Ross
  River virus)
Botulism
Brucellosis
Campylobacter infection
Chancroid
Chlamydia infection
Cholera
Cryptosporidial infection
Diphtheria
Donovanosis
Food- and water-borne illness (two or
  more related cases)
Gastroenteritis in an institution
  (residential, educational or childcare
  facility)
Giardia infection
Gonococcal infection
Haemolytic uraemic syndrome
Haemophilus influenzae type B infection
Hepatitis A
Hepatitis B
Hepatitis C
Hepatitis D
Hepatitis E
HIV infection (including AIDS)
Hydatid infection
Influenza
Legionellosis
Leprosy
Leptospirosis

Listeriosis
Lymphogranuloma venereum
Lyssavirus
Malaria
Measles
Meningococcal infection (invasive
    disease only)
Mumps
Mycobacterial infection (including
    tuberculosis)
Ornithosis
Pertussis
Plague
Pneumococcal infection
Poliomyelitis
paratyphoidosis
Q Fever
Rabies
Rickettsial infection
Rubella
Salmonella infection (including typhoid)
Shigella infection
Syphilis
Taeniasis
Tetanus
Tuberculosis
Typhoid
Typhus
Vancomycin-resistant enterocci (VRE)
Vibrio infection (including cholera)
Viral haemorrhagic fever
Yellow fever
Yersinia infection (including
plague)

Victoria
AIDS
Amoebiasis

Anthrax
Arbovirus infections
Botulism
Brucellosis
Campylobacter infection
Chlamydia infections
Chancroid
Cholera
Cryptosporidiosis
Diphtheria
Donovanosis
Food- and water-borne illness (two or
    more related cases)
Giardiasis
Gonorrhoea (all forms)
Hepatitis (viral, unspecified)
Hepatitis A
Hepatitis B
Hepatitis C
Hepatitis D
Hepatitis E
Hydatid disease
Influenza
Legionellosis
Leprosy
Leptospirosis
Listeriosis
Lymphogranuloma venereum
Malaria
Measles
Meningitis or epiglottitis due to
    Haemophilus influenzae
Meningococcal infection (meningitis or
    meningococcaemia)
Mumps
Parathyroid
Pertussis
Plague
Pneumococcal infection
Poliomyelitis

Primary amoebic meningoencephalitis
Psittacosis (ornithosis)
Q fever
Rabies
Rubella (including congenital rubella)
Salmonellosis
Shigellosis
Syphilis (all forms)
Tetanus
Tuberculosis
Typhoid and paratyphoid fevers
Typhus
Viral haemorrhagic fevers
Yellow fever
Yersiniosis

Western Australia

Adverse event following immunisation
AIDS
Amoebiasis
Amoebic meningitis
Anthrax
Arbovirus encephalitis
Barmah Forest virus infection
Brucellosis
Campylobacter infection
Chancroid (soft sore)
Chlamydia (genital infection)
Cholera
Dengue fever
Diphtheria
Donovanosis (granuloma inguinale)
Giardiasis
Gonorrhoea
Haemolytic uraemic syndrome
Haemophilus influenzae type B infection

Hepatitis A
Hepatitis B
Hepatitis C
HIV
Hydatid disease
Legionella infection
Leprosy
Leptospirosis
Malaria
Measles
Meningococcal infection
Methicillin-resistant Staphylococcus
    aureus (MRSA) infection
Mumps
Paratyphoid fever
Pertussis
Plague
Poliomyelitis
Psittacosis (ornithosis)
Q fever
Rabies
Relapsing fever
Ross River virus infection
Rubella
Salmonella infection
Scarlet fever
Schistosomiasis (Bilharzia)
Shigellosis (bacillary dysentery)
Syphilis
Tetanus
Tuberculosis (all forms)
Typhoid
Typhus (rickettsial infection)
Vibroparahaemolyticus infection
Viral haemorrhagic fevers (Crimean-
    Congo, Ebola, Lassa,
Marburg)
Yellow fever
Yersinia infection

Answers to Questions

1. My husband is going to have major surgery in a big public hospital. Is he likely to get 'golden staph' while he is there?

There is always a risk of acquiring an infection while in hospital, especially if you are elderly or very ill. The more complex the patient's operation, or the greater the number of procedures, the higher the risk. However staff members will provide all possible infection-control measures to minimise this risk.

2. I've heard there are bugs in hospitals now that eat your flesh. How long until they get into aged care?

Such organisms have been present in certain wounds, but they are not a huge concern at present.

3. Can HIV be transmitted by mosquitoes?

No.

4. Can I catch HIV from a door handle touched by a homosexual?

No.

5. Is chickenpox a sexually transmitted disease?

No, but it could be acquired during sex if there is contact with the fluid in the blisters—if the other person has not had chickenpox.

6. Is it true that shingles causes chickenpox?

No. Shingles is caused by the activation of the chickenpox virus in a person who has had chickenpox.

7. The lady in the next unit has chickenpox. To be safe, how many times do I have to wash my clothes after she has used our washing machine?

Transmission of chickenpox is via contact with the fluid in the blisters and droplets. A hot wash cycle on a shared washing machine should be adequate to prevent the transmission of the disease.

8. My son lives in the city and has been diagnosed with scabies. He is coming home and has not been treated. Are we at risk in the country?

Yes, anyone in contact with him whilst he is affected but untreated is certainly at risk.

9. One of the laundry staff caught scabies from a resident. Does that mean she wasn't washing her hands properly?

No. As well as being transmitted by direct contact, scabies can also be contracted by recently contaminated linen.

10. A resident transported in the centre's car has been diagnosed with head lice, what do we do with the car?
Vacuum it out and clean all surfaces that were in contact with the resident.

11. Can I catch meningitis from a friend at home and then take it to work?
Only if you actually acquire the condition yourself.

12. My doctor has just told me on the telephone that I am a hepatitis B carrier and to see him in three months. What do I do in the meantime, especially about my husband and children?
Make an appointment with the doctor to clarify issues and plan follow-up of contacts (including family members) for immunisation.

13. My doctor told me I was a hepatitis B carrier and that I should not even shake hands with anybody. Is this correct?
Consult your doctor again to clarify which type of hepatitis you have and how it is transmitted.

14. A person with hepatitis C has slashed himself. What do I do with the knife?
Wash the knife in hot soapy water—but ensure you wear protective gloves when doing this.

15. A person in the hostel room next to me has hepatitis C. How can I get him out of the hostel?
You can't—due to anti-discrimination legislation. Nor do you need to do so. Ring the local health department for information, you will discover that your risk of acquiring the virus is minimal.

16. A friend who I think has HIV washes his Band-Aids prior to disposal. Is that right?
It is not necessary. He is overreacting.

17. I needed a fix yesterday and the only syringe and needle available were from an HIV positive person. Do you think I will get it?
That was not a good move. I suggest you consult a GP for assessment and support.

18. I want a tattoo. Can I catch HIV this way?
Provided single-use or sterilised needles are used there is not likely to be a problem. Check with the operator about their practices.

19. I have bought a second-hand thermos and my husband is afraid of catching AIDS from it. Is this possible?

No. Just wash it in hot water and detergent before use and this will remove any micro-organisms.

20. I'm HIV positive, do I have to tell my employer?

Legally, you have no obligation to inform your employer.

21. We want to screen all our new residents for hepatitis B, hepatitis C, and HIV—just so we know if any of them are infectious. What do you think?

I think this is unnecessary. All residents must be treated the same—that is with the use of standard precautions, as if they are all infected.

22. The charge nurse says we have to use 'university precautions' when we empty pans. I left school before VCE so does it apply to me?

The proper terminology used to be 'universal', but is now 'standard precautions'. When staff members use standard precautions in their resident care it means that all body fluids of all residents are regarded as having the potential to contain transmittable organisms that might invade and cause infection or disease.

23. At our establishment we practice standard precautions, but what do we do with the linen now we have a hepatitis B carrier as a resident?

If standard precautions are properly carried out no extra care is required.

24. We have admitted our first HIV resident. Is it appropriate to use disposable cutlery and crockery?

Provided cutlery and crockery are washed properly in hot water and detergent there is no need for disposable equipment.

25. One of our residents is 79 and used to be gay. Should we test him for HIV?

As this person has been with you for a period of time, and presumably shows no symptoms, I see no point in screening for HIV.

26. Our establishment has been asked to admit an elderly woman who is HIV positive. I am not worried about the HIV but have grave concerns about the AIDS.

If you are not worried about the HIV, you need not worry about the AIDS—the preventative measures are the same. AIDS is the condition caused by the effect of HIV on the immune system.

27. Our occupational health and safety policy states that AIDS can be transmitted through unbroken skin and is very virulent this way. Is this correct?
HIV needs to leave the blood stream of an infected person and enter the blood stream of an uninfected person. Transmission would be unlikely if the skin is intact.

28. Is it true that all linen skips should be covered with drawsheets to keep the bugs in?
Bugs don't jump. If the drawsheet has contact with soiled linen it can cause contamination when removed from the skip and placed on another surface.

29. In our nursing home, the staff wear long-sleeved gowns and gloves all day, to ensure that no staff members are placed at risk of acquiring any infection. Is this appropriate?
No, this is an example of 'overkill'. The gowns can cause infection if worn for the care of more than one resident. Because it would be too expensive to wear a clean gown every time you attended a resident, it would be better to give up the gown-wearing and concentrate on your infection-control practices. Assess the risk in each task and take the appropriate action.

30. We are a nursing home and all our patients are clean. Do we really need infection-control practices in place?
Residents may be clean but infection is still possible, due to the increased susceptibility of aged residents and the likelihood of cross infection.

31. Is it true that vinegar and methylated spirits are alternatives to disinfectants?
Definitely not. Their only use is to make surfaces shine.

32. Is it appropriate to clean bench tops by spraying and wiping with gluteraldehyde?
No. This is 'overkill', and there are occupational health and safety risks involved in using the solution in this way.

33. One of our residents has 'golden staph' in a foot ulcer so we are reverse barrier nursing him in a two-bed room. The staff wear gown, gloves and mask. Is this appropriate?
The wound should be isolated, not the resident. Ensure there is always a clean dressing on the wound and that it is changed as soon as exudate shows through. The dressing must be disposed of in the infectious waste container.

34. In our establishment we soak all pans in Detsol or Safsol before the sanitiser cycle, just to make sure they are clean. Is this appropriate?

No, this is unnecessary.

35. Is it satisfactory to put instruments through a hot water disinfector then leave them soaking in sodium hypochlorite until they are required for use?

No. This method leaves the instrument at risk of contamination in the solution, and there is no guarantee that the disinfector has killed all bacteria or viruses.

36. Why is it that recapping of used needles is not recommended?

Recapping of needles is not recommended unless a single-use recapping device is used correctly. This is because of the likelihood of a needlestick injury occurring while recapping the needle.

37. Can we use a microwave oven as a steriliser?

No. There is no way of ascertaining that the required temperature for sterilisation is achieved, let alone the 'holding time', or amount of time at the required temperature.

38. I don't know how long to leave the autoclave on for. Can you advise?

Read any available technical data or gain additional information from the supplier or manufacturer.

39. Is it acceptable to seal steriliser bags with autoclave tape?

No, autoclave tape will not completely seal the bag.

40. I get dermatitis from soap. Is it all right if I don't wash my hands before doing a dressing?

No. Consult a pharmacist or dermatologist to find a product that you can use comfortably to properly clean your hands.

41. A patient in the next building had TB. Should I have a chest X-ray?

No. Prolonged contact with a person who has a productive cough is needed for you to be considered exposed.

42. To save on catheter bags the night staff leave catheters draining into urinals. Is that OK?

No. Opening what should be a closed system leaves the lumen (inside) of the catheter open to colonisation by micro-organisms. This provides an ideal environment for infection.

43. The manager says we have to re-use single-use insulin syringes. We wash them in hot soapy water but I still don't feel right about it. What do you think?
Single-use means single use. There is no way of ensuring that the syringes have been adequately decontaminated.

44. We're supposed to wear goggles when sluicing linen, but I don't because some of the staff are gay and I'm worried about catching something. What do you suggest?
Sluicing of linen is an infection-control and occupational health-and-safety risk. If you must sluice, appropriate protective clothing (including goggles) must be worn. Other staff members' lifestyles should not affect your infection-control practices.

45. We soak all the enteral feeding giving sets together in sodium hypochlorite. Is that enough to kill the germs?
If the equipment is kept separate from other giving sets, and returned to the same person, washing in hot water and detergent is adequate. Soaking all residents' sets together will lead to cross-infection.

46. The labels have come off all the drums in the cleaners' room and I washed the floor with shampoo by mistake. Will it kill the germs anyway?
Shampoo is just that—for use on hair. Technical information sheets will show you that the properties are different. In addition, the shampoo might make the floor slippery.

47. The unit manager says we have to wipe everything with bleach, but it's taking the colour out of the furnishings. Is there an alternative?
Bleach should not be used as a cleaning agent as it does not have cleaning properties.

48. I'm too short to reach the high shelves with my duster. Is it that important?
Dust on shelves must be removed as a build up can cause dust drifting to other areas.

49. When the linen is delivered it's still damp. The laundry contractor dumps it on the ground outside the kitchen. Should we make him bring it into the foyer?
Clean linen should arrive dry and be treated in such a way that it does not come into contact with contaminated surfaces.

50. Why can't we use Betadine packs on wound cavities any more? They used to work well.

Research has shown that Betadine used to pack cavities may cause toxicity.

51. The union says it's not my job to bring the milk inside when it's delivered to our nursing home. The residents like it warm anyway. Is that a problem?

Milk that is not refrigerated may grow organisms and cause illness. Talk to your manager about how the milk can be properly stored.

52. We throw all the rubbish in to the skip. The residents in the room beside it complain about the smell, but will they catch anything from it?

The residents will not catch anything unless they come into contact with the waste. But aesthetically it is unacceptable.

53. On week nights I have to clean the pan room before I give out the suppers. Is this acceptable?

Provided you practise good handwashing and good housekeeping, the risk is reduced. It would, however, be better to give out the suppers, and then clean the pan room.

54. We got a new air conditioning system last summer and now every one is getting colds. Could it be Legionnaire's disease?

No, I think it is likely to be coincidental.

55. There are lots of stray cats behind the hostel, and the kitchen staff leave milk out for them. Will any germs get into the food?

The practice should be discouraged, but at least ensure the animals do not enter the kitchen and that staff maintain good personal hygiene.

56. We had an outbreak of gastroenteritis at work last winter, and even the staff became sick. The DON said it couldn't be the food because the kitchen staff are very clean. Would this be right?

When there is an outbreak of gastroenteritis, both food storage and staff food-handling practices must be reviewed. The real question is: Are the personal hygiene standards and housekeeping practices of the kitchen staff acceptable? Both should be investigated.

Glossary

Glossary

Abscess
A localised collection of pus formed as a result of infection and inflammation.

Antibiotic
A chemical agent with the ability to interfere with the development of a living organism or destroy it.

Antibody
An antigen-neutralising substance formed by the body tissues in response to a challenge by an introduced foreign protein.

Antigen
A substance that, when introduced into the body, stimulates the production of antibodies.

Antiseptic
A substance that inhibits the growth and reproduction of micro-organisms when applied to a surface.

Asepsis
1. The prevention of contamination by the exclusion or destruction of micro-organisms.
2. The state of being free from living pathogenic organisms.

Aseptic technique
A procedural technique, beginning with a clinical hand-wash that aims to exclude micro-organisms from the sterile field.

Bacillus
A rod-shaped bacterium, commonly known as a germ.

Bacteraemia
The presence of bacteria in the blood.

Bacteria
Plural of bacterium.

Bacterium
A microscopic organism capable of colonising a host and causing illness.

Bioburden
Contaminating body tissue debris.

Biocides
A physical or chemical agent that is capable of killing micro-organisms.

Body fluids
Fluid substances that come from the human body, including blood, saliva, semen, sputum, vomit, amniotic fluid, cerebrospinal fluid (CSF), pleural or peritoneal fluids, synovial fluid, urine, and faeces.

Body substance isolation
An infection-control practice that aims to prevent contact with any body substance, whether infected or not (see standard precautions).

Carrier
A person who harbours and excretes disease-producing organisms without necessarily suffering from the associated disease.

Cleaning
Mechanical removal of surface contaminants, such as bioburden and dust.

Colonisation
The presence of micro-organisms in the body without sign of infection.

Contamination
The introduction of micro-organisms to the body or an inanimate object.

Cross infection
A means of spreading infection from an infected person to an uninfected person.

Culture
A laboratory-produced growth of micro-organisms, for study and identification purposes.

Decontamination
The cleaning and disinfection of used articles in order to make them safe to handle.

Detergent
A chemical cleaning agent that suspends contaminants and enables them to be easily removed.

Direct contact
A method of spreading disease from a source to a host by physical contact between the two.

Disinfection
The process of killing or removing micro-organism, with the possible exception of bacterial spores.

Endogenous infection
Self-infection caused by micro-organisms normally carried without sign of illness.

Epidemic
An increase, above expected incidence, of an organism or disease.

Exogenous infection
An infection, or cross-infection, originating outside the body.

Exudate
A fluid with cellular debris that escapes from the tissues as a result of inflammation or infection.

Flagging
The outmoded practice of using a marker on specimen containers to identify specimens that pose a specific infection risk.

Fomites
Inanimate objects, other than food, which when contaminated act as a reservoir of micro-organisms.

Gram-positive/Gram-negative
A method of classifying micro-organisms by staining with a purple dye called 'Gram's stain'. Those micro-organisms that take up the stain are said to be Gram-positive, whereas those that do not are Gram-negative.

Host
A living organism, such as a human, which harbours micro-organisms.

Immunisation
The process of increasing resistance to certain infectious diseases by deliberately provoking an immune response.

Immunosuppression
An individual's immune response is suppressed or prevented due to inadequate white cell production.

Incubation period
The period of time between exposure to an organism and the appearance of signs or symptoms of illness.

Infection
The deposition and harmful multiplication of micro-organisms in tissues or on the surfaces of the body, followed by signs and symptoms of clinical illness.

Infectious disease
The harmful result of infection.

Infectious period
The period of time during an infectious disease when the pathogen can be transmitted to another host.

Inflammation
The body's defensive reaction to tissue injury (increased blood flow and capillary permeability), which destroys or dilutes the injuring agent, or walls-off the injury.

Mantoux skin test
A subcutaneous injection of tuberculin which, when inspected for a reaction three days later, indicates whether the person has had contact with the tubercule bacillus.

Microbe
A micro-organism, especially pathogenic bacteria.

Micro-organisms
Microscopic organisms, including bacteria, fungi, and viruses, capable of infecting a host.

Normal flora
Micro-organisms which normally colonise specific body sites.

Non-touch technique
Avoiding contact with body fluids or broken skin and mucous membranes while performing a procedure.

Nosocomial infection
Infection acquired by staff or residents in a health care institution.

Notifiable diseases
Diseases that must be reported to the health department.

Opportunistic organisms
Micro-organisms which normally have little or no pathogenic activity.

Glossary

Pathogen
A micro-organism capable of causing disease.

Pus
Thick fluid usually yellow in colour, composed of bacteria, white blood cells, necrotic (dead) tissue, and other products of tissue breakdown.

Resistant organism
A micro-organism that is not affected by a given antibiotic.

Safe sex
The use of a protective barrier during sexual intercourse (usually a condom) to avoid contact with a sexual partner's body fluids.

Septicaemia
Systemic disease associated with the presence of pathogenic microorganisms in the blood stream.

Sluicing
The practice of using high-pressure water to irrigate solid particles of body fluids, such as faeces, from linen before laundering.

Spores, bacterial
Thick-walled cells formed by specific Gram-positive bacteria during their inactive stage. Spores are resistant to heat and chemical destruction and may survive for long periods.

Standard precautions
The precautions that staff take to avoid contact with any blood and body fluids, regardless of the source. The precautions involve using barrier techniques, such as masking, hand-washing, or protective clothing.

Sterilisation
The process of killing and/or removing all micro-organisms including bacterial spores, from inanimate objects.

Transient micro-organisms
Micro-organisms not normally found at a particular site but readily removed by normal washing.

Tuberculin
A sterile, non-contagious liquid derived from the tubercule bacillus, used in a Mantoux test to diagnose tuberculosis.

Unprotected sexual intercourse
Either heterosexual or homosexual sexual intercourse, where there is no barrier (usually a condom) to direct contact between the penis and the receptive tissue of the other partner.

Universal precautions
See standard precautions.

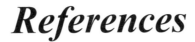

References

References

Introduction

1. Bennett J and Brachman P (eds) (1998): Hospital Infections (Fourth edition). Boston: Little, Brown and Company.

2. Victorian Government Department of Human Services (1998): *Infection Control in Victorian Public Hospitals*. Melbourne: Department of Human Services p. 1.

3. Commonwealth Department of Health and Family Services (1997): *Draft Standards for Aged Care Facilities*. Canberra: Australian Government Publishing Service. Also available at: www.health.gov.au/acc/manuals.

4. Commonwealth Department of Health and Family Services (1997): *Draft Standards for Aged Care Facilities*. Canberra: Australian Government Publishing Service. Also available at: www.health.gov.au/acc/manuals.

5. Australian Health-Care Associates and Commonwealth Department of Health and Family Services (1997): *Aged Care Structural Reform Strategy: Standards and Workbook*. Melbourne: Australian Health-Care Associates p. 10.

Chapter 1

1. Victorian Government Department of Human Services (1998): *Infection Control in Victorian Public Hospitals*. Melbourne: Department of Human Services p. 1.

2. Victorian Government Department of Human Services (1998): *Infection Control in Victorian Public Hospitals*. Melbourne: Department of Human Services p. 1.

3. Standing Committee on Infection Control (1992): *Guidelines for Control of Infection in Hospitals and Other Health Care Institutions*. Melbourne: Health Department Victoria p. 6.

4. Standing Committee on Infection Control (1992): *Guidelines for Control of Infection in Hospitals and Other Health Care Institutions*. Melbourne: Health Department Victoria p. 8.

5. Castle M (1980): *Hospital Infection Control: Principles and Practice*. New York: Wiley Medical pp. 56–58.

6. Castle M (1980): Hospital Infection Control: Principles and Practice. New York: Wiley Medical p. 41.

7. Johnson and Johnson Medical Pty Ltd (1992): Hands up and be counted. (Video recording).

8. National Health & Medical Research Council and Australian National Council on AIDS (1996): Infection Control in the Health Care Setting: Guidelines for the Prevention of Transmission of Infectious Diseases. Canberra: Australian Government Publishing Service p. 11.

9. Department of Human Services (1998): Infection Control Guidelines for the Management of Patients with Methicillin-resistant Staphylococcus aureus (MRSA) and Vancomycin-resistant Enterococci (VRE) in Long-Term Care Facilities (LTCF). Information sheet. Melbourne: Department of Human Services.

10. Bogle B and Bogle G (1997): Acquiring Vancomycin-resistant Enterococcus (VRE). *Advance* 9:18.

Chapter 2

1. National Health and Medical Research Council and Australian National Council on AIDS (1996): *Infection Control in the Health Care Setting: Guidelines for the Prevention of Transmission of Infectious Diseases.* Canberra: Australian Government Publishing Service p. 120.

2. National Health and Medical Research Council (1997): *The Australian Immunisation Handbook* (Sixth edition). Canberra: Australian Government Publishing Service p. 39.

3. Australian National Council on AIDS (1992): Management of Exposure to Blood/Body Fluids Contaminated With Blood, including Needle stick/Sharps Injuries with a Potential for HIV or Other Blood Borne Infections. *Bulletin*: No. 16.

4. Department of Human Services (1997): *Occupational Exposure to HIV Infection.* Information sheet. Melbourne: Department of Human Services.

5. Health and Community Services (1994): *TB. Be Aware: Eliminating Tuberculosis, a Strategy for Victoria.* Health and Community Services Resource Kit. Melbourne: Health and Community Services.

Chapter 3

1. Health and Community Services (1994): TB. Be Aware: Eliminating Tuberculosis, a Strategy for Victoria. Health and Community Services Resource Kit. Melbourne: Health and Community Services.

2. Health and Community Services (1994): *Food Premises Code* (Second edition). Melbourne: Health and Community Services.

3. Australian Government Publishing Service (1995): *Food Service Hygiene and Cleaning* (Fourth edition). Canberra: Australian Government Printing Service.

4. Department of Human Services (1998): *Infection Control Guidelines for the Management of Patients with Methicillin-resistant Staphylococcus aureus (MRSA) and Vancomycin-resistant Enterococci (VRE) in Long-Term Care Facilities (LTCF).* Information Sheet. Melbourne: Department of Human Services.

5. Stucke V (1993): *Microbiology for Nurses: Applications to Patient Care.* London: Baillière Tindall.

Chapter 4

1. National Health and Medical Research Council and Australian National Council on AIDS (1996): *Infection Control in the Health Care Setting: Guidelines for the Prevention of Transmission of Infectious Diseases.* Canberra: Australian Government Publishing Service.

2. Johnson and Johnson Medical Pty Ltd (1992): Hands up and be counted. (Video recording).

3. National Health and Medical Research Council and Australian National Council on AIDS (1996): *Infection Control in the Health Care Setting: Guidelines for the Prevention of Transmission of Infectious Diseases.* Canberra: Australian Government Publishing Service.

4. Standards Australia (1992): *Non-reusable Containers for the Collection of Sharp Medical Items Used in Health Care Areas (AS 4031–1992).* Sydney: Standards Australia.

5. National Health and Medical Research Council and Australian National Council on AIDS (1996): *Infection Control in the Health Care Setting: Guidelines for the Prevention of Transmission of Infectious Diseases.* Canberra: Australian Government Publishing Service.

6. Castle M (1980): *Hospital Infection Control: Principles and Practice.* New York: Wiley Medical p. 73.

Chapter 5

1. National Health and Medical Research Council and Australian National Council on AIDS (1996): *Infection Control in the Health Care Setting: Guidelines for the Prevention of Transmission of Infectious Diseases.* Canberra: Australian Government Publishing Service.

2. Adapted from: National Health and Medical Research Council and Australian National Council on AIDS (1996): *Infection Control in the Health Care Setting: Guidelines for the Prevention of Transmission of Infectious Diseases.* Canberra: Australian Government Publishing Service p. 41.

184
References

3. Standards Australia (2003): *Code of Practice for Cleaning, Disinfecting and Sterilizing Reusable Medical and Surgical Instruments and Equipment, and Maintenance of Associated Environments in Health Care Facilities (AS/NZS 4187: 2003)*. Sydney: Standards Australia.

4. Castle M (1980): *Hospital Infection Control: Principles and practice*. New York: Wiley Medical. Chapter 6.

5. Bennett J and Brachman P (eds) (1998): *Hospital Infections* (Fourth edition). Boston: Little, Brown and Company.

6. OHS/WorkCover Advisory Committee (1996): *Guidelines For The Use Of Gluteraldehyde In The Health Industry*. Melbourne: Department of Human Services.

7. Bennett J and Brachman P (eds) (1998): *Hospital Infections* (Fourth edition). Boston: Little, Brown and Company p. 81f.

8. Standards Australia (2003): *Code of Practice for Cleaning, Disinfecting and Sterilizing Reusable Medical and Surgical Instruments and Equipment, and Maintenance of Associated Environments in Health Care Facilities (AS/NZS 4187: 2003)*. Sydney: Standards Australia.

9. Health and Community Services (1994): *Infection Control Guidelines For Procedures Involving Penetration of Skin, Mucous Membrane and/or Other Tissue*. Information sheet. Melbourne: Health and Community Services.

10. Standards Australia (1994): *Code of Practice for Cleaning, Disinfecting and Sterilizing Reusable Medical and Surgical Instruments and Equipment, and Maintenance of Associated Environments in Health Care Facilities (AS/NZS 4187: 2003)*. Sydney: Standards Australia.

11. Health and Community Services (1994): *Infection Control Guidelines For Procedures Involving Penetration of Skin, Mucous Membrane and/or Other Tissue*. Information sheet. Melbourne: Health and Community Services.

12. Sussman G (1994): The use of antiseptics in wounds. Melbourne. Wound Foundation of Australia.

13. Health and Community Services (1994): *Infection Control Guidelines For Procedures Involving Penetration of Skin, Mucous Membrane and/or Other Tissue*. Information sheet. Melbourne: Health and Community Services.

14. Victorian Medical Postgraduate Foundation Inc. (1996–1997): *Antibiotic Guidelines* (9th edition). Melbourne: Victorian Medical Postgraduate Foundation Inc.

15. Department of Human Services (1998): *Infection Control Guidelines for the Management of Patients with Methicillin Resistant Staphylococcus Aureus (MRSA) and Vancomycin Resistant Enterococci (VRE) in Long Term Care Facilities (LTCF)*. Information sheet. Melbourne: Department of Human Services p. 2.

16. Health Department Victoria (1989): *Guidelines for the Control of Legionnaires' Disease*. Melbourne: Health Department Victoria.

17. Department of Human Services (1997): *Protocol for Management and Prevention of Outbreaks of Infectious Diseases in Homes for the Elderly*. Information Sheet. Melbourne: Department of Human Services.

18. Health and Community Services (1994): *Food Premises Code* (Second edition). Melbourne: Health and Community Services.

19. Australian Government Publishing Service (1995): *Food Service Hygiene and Cleaning* (Fourth edition). Canberra: Australian Government Printing Service.

20. Department of Human Services (1997): *Food Safety Programs for the Food Service Sector*. Melbourne. Victorian Government Department of Human Services.

21. Standards Australia (2000): *Laundry Practice (AS/NZS 4146: 2000)*. Sydney: Standards Australia.

22. Standards Australia (2000): *Laundry Practice (AS/NZS 4146: 2000)*. Sydney: Standards Australia.

23. National Health and Medical Research Council (1988): *National Guidelines for the Management of Clinical and Related Wastes*. Canberra: Australian Government Publishing Service.

24. National Health and Medical Research Council and Australian National Council on AIDS (1996): *Infection Control in the Health Care Setting: Guidelines for the prevention of transmission of infectious diseases*. Canberra: Australian Government Publishing Service p. 26.

25. Australian/New Zealand Management of Clinical and Related Wastes (AS/NZS 3816: 1999 p. 8.)

Chapter 6

1. Ell M and Ell J (1991): *Quality Assurance Demystified*. Melbourne: Rolls Printing.

2. Commonwealth Department of Health and Family Services (1997): *Draft Standards for Aged Care Facilities*. Canberra: Australian Government Publishing Service. Also available at: www.health.gov.au/acc/manuals.

3. Australian Health-care Associates and Commonwealth Department of Health and Family Services (1997): *Aged Care Structural Reform Strategy: Standards and Workbook*. Melbourne: Australian Health-Care Associates.

4. Australian Health-Care Associates and Commonwealth Department of Health and Family Services (1997): *Aged Care Structural Reform Strategy: Standards and Workbook*. Melbourne: Australian Health-Care Associates.

5. National Health and Medical Research Council and Australian National Council on AIDS (1996): *Infection Control in the Health Care Setting: Guidelines for the Prevention of Transmission of Infectious Diseases*. Canberra: Australian Government Publishing Service.

6. Victorian Medical Postgraduate Foundation Inc. (1996–97): *Antibiotic Guidelines* (9th edition). Melbourne: Victorian Medical Postgraduate Foundation Inc.

7. Department of Human Services (1997): *Protocol for Management and Prevention of Outbreaks of Infectious Diseases in Homes for the Elderly*. Information Sheet. Melbourne: Department of Human Services.

8. Garner J S, Jarvis W R, Emori T G, Horan T C, Hughes J M (1988): CDC *Definitions for Nosocomial Infections*. Atlanta Georgia: Centre for Disease Control.

9. McGeer A, Campbell B, Emoi T, et al. (1991): Definitions of infection for surveillance in long-term care facilities. *American Journal of Infection Control* 19 (1).

Chapter 7

1. Stucke V (1993): Microbiology for Nurses: Applications to Patient Care. London: Baillière Tindall.

2. Department of Human Services (1997): The Blue Book: Guidelines for the Control of Infectious Diseases. Melbourne: Department of Human Services.

3. South Australian Health Commission (1992): You've got what? Control of Infectious Diseases in Children and Adults. Adelaide: South Australian Health Commission.

4. Health Department Victoria (1989): *Guidelines for the Control of Legionnaires' Disease*. Melbourne. Health Department Victoria.

5. National Occupational Health and Safety Commission (1993): HIV and the Workplace: *Information for Health Workers and Others at Risk*. Canberra: Australian Government Printer.

Index